Reflections from the Emergency Room

I didn't know if I was in heaven or hell, but something was definitely not right! I am the picture of health! What am I doing here? Sue called Fred and Melanie and they arrived within 24 hours. Hmm, this must be serious!

"*Hi Dad, how are you feeling?*" asked Melissa our youngest.

How was I feeling! Like I had been run over by a freight train and left for dead! What in the world just happened to me?

The doctor took one look at me and said, "*Something is seriously wrong, we don't know what it is yet, look at your hand next to mine*." He rolled his palm up next to mine and I finally saw what everyone had been talking about. His palm was a healthy pink and mine was a grayish yellow.

I nicknamed myself the Rabbit Man while being transfused with Rabbit Serum designed to suppress my immune system. This was supposed to allow my platelets and other vital blood cells the opportunity to grow normally. I had been diagnosed with Aplastic Anemia, a rare blood disorder that occurs when the bone marrow stops making enough healthy blood cells.

From one of the first mothers to visit the website.

"Our hematologist seems to think our daughter may have AA but has not diagnosed her yet. She has a bone marrow test on Friday morning. I have been reading up since he talked to us this morning to try and educate myself. Our doctor mentioned this is a worst-case scenario so I am a little interested as to what that means. He would not go into specifics with us today because he wants to see all the tests. Her hemoglobin was at 2.1 last night so they rushed her to PICU. It all has happened so fast. I am praying often and will continue researching. My daughter is 2 months old so the doctor is very confused as she is very young. I would like to get on a mailing list for news about this disease and also any advice or good questions to ask the doctors would be appreciated. Thanks."

Aplastic Anemia & Autoimmune Diseases

Heal Your Body With A Personal Wellness Plan

Bruce Lande

Second Edition
Update Contact Information

Holden Beach, North Carolina

Aplastic Anemia & Autoimmune Diseases
Heal Your Body with a Personal Wellness Plan

By **Bruce Lande**
Published by:
Bruce Lande
507 Ocean Boulevard West
Holden Beach, NC
http://apasticcentral.org

All rights reserved. No part of this book may be reproduced or transmitted in any form or by any means, electronic or mechanical, including photocopying, recording or by any information storage and retrieval system, without written permission from the author, except for the inclusion of brief quotations in review.

Unattributed quotations are by Bruce Lande
Copyright 2002 by Bruce Lande

ISBN, print Ed.   1-9781793492418

First Printing 2002
Second Printing 2019

Printed in the United States of America
Library of Congress Cataloging-in-Publication Data
Lande, Bruce

Aplastic anemia & autoimmune diseases: heal your body with a personal wellness plan/Bruce Lande – 1st ed. P.cm.

Includes bibliographical references (p.) and index ISBN 1-xxxxx-xxx-x

1. Aplastic anemia & autoimmune diseases –United States. I. Title
2. Health
3. Alternative healing

About the Author

Caution - The author is not a medical professional. This book is a guide to help you understand more about your illness and present alternative methods for healing your body. Please contact your caretakers before using any of the information presented.

In January of 2001, Bruce Lande was informed that he had less than six months to live and after evaluating the recommended treatment protocols and the alternative treatments available for Aplastic Anemia, decided to develop a website to host his research. The website allowed him to be in contact with many other people who had Aplastic Anemia and similar Autoimmune Related Illnesses.

He soon realized that very little had been written on these illnesses by a patient. Although there are numerous scientific studies and clinical trials, no one appeared to have told the story in a manner that was easily understood by the patient. The daily struggles, the emotional swings, the feelings of hopelessness were not documented.

Beginning in August of 2001, Bruce and his wife of over 30 years formulated "A Personal Wellness Plan" that has resulted in him not only extending his life beyond original expectations but has offered him a whole new quality of life.

In this book, Bruce describes Aplastic Anemia in terms that everyone can understand. He then describes the conventional treatments available. Finally, he offers you the elements of the Personal Wellness Plan that he believes can help virtually everyone, whether ill or not, develop and maintain a better quality of life.

As of January 9, 2019, 18 years later, Bruce is in full remission and living a completely normal life. Follow updates and plans for a full third edition and sequel at http://aplasticcentral.org.

Dedication

To Sue and our family and to Gay who encouraged me to get back in the game.

Acknowledgements

Without the incredible kindness of strangers and the unbelievable support of Sue, our daughters and their husbands, Sue's family and our friends, I would not be here today.

Special thanks also to the many people who cared for me during my illness and the many participants at http://aplasticcentral.org.

Preface to Second Edition and Note to the Reader

The second edition is primarily to update contact information and to replace all references to aplasticcentral.com with the new website rename aplasticcentral.org. As I write this preface to the second edition, I am updating the website and beginning work on the sequel to the original book. If you would like to be notified when the next edition is available, please go to the contact us section of the new website.

If you want to skip my story and "cut to the chase", please fast forward to the chapter on Aplastic Anemia. If, on the other hand, you are interested in how we developed our strategy and how we dealt with the many ups and downs associated with a chronic illness, begin, as they say, at the beginning.

If you have an autoimmune disorder or cancer, you may want to start with the chapter entitled AA, Autoimmune Disorders and Cancer and then return to the beginning.

Aplastic Anemia and Myelodysplastic Syndromes are both precursors to leukemia and that means that unless we beat this thing that we have now, we will shortly be battling cancer. While I was writing the book, several people that I knew died of cancer and I urged them to consider the alternative program before it was too late.

Most of the treatments set forth in this book are very inexpensive (except my trip to EHCD) and are based on items available from nature or at your local grocery store. Helping your body heal itself will not be accomplished with any magic potions. It does require a dedicated effort, time, patience and a new way of thinking.

This book is designed for the sole purpose of helping the reader develop a Personal Wellness Plan. It is to be used in conjunction with a doctor or other health care professional. It is sold with the understanding that the neither the author nor any other participants in the preparation of the book, except as noted, have medical training. The wellness plan and other recommendations in the book should be thoroughly discussed with a medical professional before use.

It is not the purpose of this book to reprint all the information that is available on Aplastic Anemia or any of the other illnesses discussed. It is designed to complement the other sources of information that are available. The reader is advised to read additional information on alternative treatments, holistic healing and the diseases themselves before proceeding with a wellness plan. Learn as much as you can about your illness and tailor your plan to fit your own personal situation.

In no way does this book, the author's website or any other materials produced by the author claim to provide a cure for the diseases discussed. The author has used the wellness plan; alternative treatments and a holistic healing program to alter his own lifestyle. He believes that the approaches described have allowed him to extend and enrich his quality of life, but the ultimate purpose of this book is to educate, not provide a get well quick scheme.

Every effort has been made to make this book as complete and accurate as possible. However, there may be mistakes. The book should therefore be used as a guide and not the ultimate source of information on the diseases or remedies discussed.

Foreword

We all know about diseases such as cancer, diabetes, and heart disease. For decades, countless books and articles have been written documenting research and hypotheses for dealing with these common diseases, for which a quick search on the Internet will reveal thousands of hits. Yet, in October of 1999, when I was diagnosed with aplastic anemia (AA), there were far fewer links on the Internet providing information on aplastic anemia. The amount of medical articles in the field of hematology available to the public on the subject of aplastic anemia was scant.

How was I to survive this disease or even make intelligent decisions regarding treatment when so little information was available? No friends, family or acquaintances had even heard of aplastic anemia. Even my own hematologist said, "I'll get back to you after I look up the treatment protocol for aplastic anemia." What kind of a disease was this so that my doctor had to "look up" the treatment? Is it that uncommon? As days passed, I continued to be more and more perplexed with tests and test results. What did all these tests mean?

Like other patients, only through hours of searching and reading was I able to piece together the information I needed to understand my condition and my options. Doctors gave some answers to my many questions, but I felt that they were as confused as I was. How much easier it would have been if all the information had been in one place!

In 2001, I discovered Bruce Lande's website, http://www.aplasticcentral.org/. As his website grew, it filled a tremendous void. Bruce's talent and obsession made it possible to track his progress, communicate with other AA patients, and follow analysis of medical and non-medical methods for dealing with this mysterious and devastating disease.

It is incredible how he was able to keep up with it all and also cope with our mutual condition. Bruce utilized his computer knowledge to reach out and unite other AA patients suffering in obscurity. He searched for AA patients throughout the world via the Internet to share information and support for AA. His efforts resulted in Aplastic Anemia Central, the largest, most informed Internet site for AA patients to learn and network together. Through many thousands of hours of research, Bruce compiled anything and everything he could find pertaining to AA and has made it available, completely free, to anyone in need.

Bruce's book, Aplastic Anemia and Autoimmune Diseases, is truly a public service to those of us searching for a quick guide to AA and other autoimmune diseases. In his (300+#) page, information-filled book, he discusses medical research, statistics, treatment options, and his own powerful personal experience. He delves into the physical aspects of AA and divulges his emotional defeats and triumphs.

In addition to cataloging the currently available medical research and treatments for AA, Bruce has included a section dedicated to various alternative methods of treatment. Treatments discussed include natural, non-toxic approaches to dealing with AA and other degenerative diseases. He has found natural treatment to be effective with his aplastic anemia. He explains and draws analogies to bodily functions to help readers understand.

Lastly, Aplastic Anemia and Autoimmune Diseases is a tribute to all the family, friends, and caretakers of AA sufferers. The experiences he shares regarding the care he was given is a reflection of the experiences of all of us who suffer from AA, both patients, and family and friends. We have family members, friends, and caretakers who also spent countless, emotionally filled hours helping us cope and survive our disease. You will feel his trying personal struggle, but you will also laugh with his great sense of humor.

If you or a loved one has suffered from AA, then I trust that Bruce shares experiences that reflect your own. His story gives a glimpse of not only the turmoil endured by the patients, but of the struggles endured by closest caretakers and supporters. Aplastic Anemia and Autoimmune Diseases is a must read for both AA patients and caretakers alike. It is a valuable addition to your arsenal of knowledge for your use in conquering aplastic anemia.

Marla Brown,

California, 2003
VSAA 10/99 Aplastic Anemia Survivor and Mentor to Many Others who Survived

Chapter 1 Triage

A Visit to the ER

"Hello Bruce, my name is Dr. Jeff Kirshner and I will be taking care of you while you are in the hospital. We already know that you have a serious blood disorder - It may or may not be leukemia. If you want to hope for something, hope it is Leukemia because we know how to treat Leukemia today. It is not as serious a disease as it was in Brian Piccolo's day.

Right now our job is to get you through the night and we will nail down the diagnosis tomorrow. You are in desperate need of blood and platelets and the Syracuse Blood Bank is out of your blood type. We are waiting for your transfusions to come from Rochester and there is a very real risk they may be closing the Thruway because of the blizzard. "

Say again! Was he talking to me? And what was this about not making it through the night? Having driven the New York State Thruway in a white out, I knew what it could be like. I was desperately looking around for some help. My wife Sue was looking at me with the same look she had on her face when our beloved Tasha died in her arms.

Melissa's look was not much better. She was the youngest of our three daughters and my partner in our computer business. What was happening here? Hey, wait just a minute - being sick was not part of my plan. There was a business to run and somebody had to be in Albany tomorrow to finish an installation.

My mind was in overdrive - Why exactly would one wish for Leukemia of all things! Leukemia kills people. I had never been sick more than a day or two in my life. Surrounded by my wife and one of our three daughters in a cramped triage room at Community General Hospital, I began to worry about how they would cope with me gone. - For the first time in my life, my own mortality seemed very real; sure it would happen someday - but in my 80's, not in my 50's.

I didn't know if I was in heaven or hell, but something was definitely not right! I am the picture of health! What was I doing here? Wow, this must be serious, Sue called Fred and Melanie and they arrived within 24 hours. "Hi Dad, how are you feeling?" asked Melissa, my partner in the web business. How was I feeling! Like I had been run over by a freight train and left for dead! What in the world just happened to me?

My Dad died at 54 and my mother at 63 so I had at least considered the possibility of a premature death. But Dad was a three pack a day smoker and I had recently endured a colonoscopy to head off the colon cancer that prematurely claimed my mother.

Dad had Hodgkin's disease in his 30's back before chemotherapy and he once told me how painful a Bone Marrow Biopsy was back then. My first biopsy to determine a proper diagnosis and prognosis was scheduled for the next day.

What happens after tonight? Will there even be a tomorrow? My life now depended on a courier delivering a life-saving parcel from Rochester - normally only an hour away and it had already been over two hours. Strangely enough, there was very little fear of death. There was more concern over what would happen to Sue and our family.

* * * * *

This concern for others had not always been part of my personal agenda. Over thirty years ago on an equally snowy day in Central New York, Sue and I were married in a quaint little country church in Lafayette, NY.

We had only known each other since July of the same year, but she stole my heart from the very beginning. She declined two of my proposals before finally relenting. From that moment on, my life as a self-centered teen-ager came to an end.

A short time later, we were living "on the economy" in the Cold War divided city of Berlin, Germany. Our lives quickly changed from that of blissful newly-weds to young, frightened parents in a strange far-away land when Sue gave birth to the first of our three daughters. Until then, responsibility had been only a vague term to me. I suddenly found myself the breadwinner for our budding little family of three.

My thoughts were bouncing back and forth between previous life altering events and my present predicament so fast I could barely keep things straight in my own mind. I returned to that cold winter night in Berlin when our oldest daughter, Michelle was born. The Air Force offered virtually no support to married enlisted men back then. Busses and the subway were our only means of transportation, so a neighbor's car became our maternity transport.

That was the first time I remember being in a hospital. Now, nearly thirty years to the day later, frantic calls were going out to Michelle and Melanie, our middle daughter. Melissa lives close by and was at her Mother's side as the doctor delivered his frightening news.

My mind flashed to another frantic event in the Pediatric Emergency Unit of the Upstate Medical Center. Our middle daughter Melanie was strapped to a "papoose board". She had been locked in this position for several hours and was in a full state of panic. Her boyfriend, Adam was a year older and apparently had been taken to the regular Emergency Room. Melanie was crying because she was sure that Adam was dead. The last she had seen him, he was unconscious, bleeding from his head in his parent's demolished car.

* * * * *

I returned to the present and wondered who would take care of our little family. They are all grown now and on their own, but once you become a father, your concerns never really go away. Melissa and Sue are heavily dependent on the website development business I had started after working for a major corporation the last ten years.

We had invested well over $100,000 of our savings to start the business and our net worth had plummeted with the drop in tech stocks and the recession-mired economy. Right now, however, we seemed to have a more pressing problem on our hands than whether or not the DOW would recover. My illness and the prospect of a premature death had now taken center stage in our lives.

* * * * *

The courier completed his life saving trip from Rochester to Syracuse in the middle of what was hailed the "Storm of the Century". The New York State Thruway had been closed but the driver somehow managed to make the normally one hour drive in just under three hours in time to save my life.

He arrived at 2:15 AM on January 10, 2001 and the first of many life-saving transfusions was administered. He delivered one unit of platelets and two units of packed red blood cells. At the time of my admission, my platelet count was just under 3,000, white blood cell count was 1,500 and my hemoglobin was 9. The normal counts for an average sized adult male are 300,000 for platelets, 6,000 for white blood cells and 15 for hemoglobin.

I later learned that even a small cut could have resulted in my death since the platelets were so few in number. Such a small number of platelets would have been unable to stop any significant bleeding and I would have literally bled to death while waiting for help.

Platelets are the components in our blood responsible for clotting. Red blood cells deliver oxygen from the heart to the other organs of the body and return the carbon dioxide to our heart for recycling. A normal adult has ten pints of blood that circulate around the body in blood vessels that if fully stretched could circle the earth two and one half times.

The Bone Marrow produces between four and five billion Red Blood Cells or "Erythrocytes" per hour and they last an average of four months. The marrow produces White Blood Cells or "Lymphocytes" which fight infection, Platelets or "Thrombocytes" that aid in clotting and Plasma, which is the water and protein component of the blood.

In addition to the concerns of blood loss and platelets, I began to understand why my stamina had been so low for so long. It was a significant effort to walk up a small flight of stairs because my blood stream was unable to deliver the oxygen necessary to nourish my leg muscles.

About two weeks prior I had experienced a "fainting spell" in which my whole left side went numb. At the time, I was carrying boxes up and down a long flight of stairs in a dusty old warehouse in Batavia, NY. It was a struggle, as I had to stop and grab the wall for support about every seven steps. It was a major sign of something seriously amiss with my health that I should have acted on.

The building had forty-foot high ceilings and smelled as though it had been a cold storage warehouse in one of its previous lives. It was now home to ARAmatic Refreshment Services, one of our best customers. Fulfilling a promise to Art Darrow, the owner, I was determined to get this, the fourth of its four New York branches online before the end of the year.

Computers had been at the center of my life long before most of the world knew input from output. The first system I ever touched literally filled a room. It was an IBM 360 with the unbelievable capacity of 64 kilobytes of memory! We fed these funny little punch cards into a tray that gobbled them up, sometimes quite literally so that you always wanted to have an extra deck of JCL - Job Control Language - available as your back up.

The machine would then sputter and lights would flash and in an awesome display of power, it would re-calculate the amount of money 1000's of bank customers owed the bank. A process that today could be done on my laptop in a matter of seconds took most of an eight-hour shift.

I began my "real" work life as a computer operator and then graduated to selling computers for a now defunct company called Digital Equipment. Computers like the one we sold for nearly one million dollars in the eighties are now available at your local Radio Shack for just under six hundred American dollars and they'll probably throw in a web cam so you can have a live videoconference with your grandchildren.

* * * * *

So here I was in this tiny antiseptic smelling room with a huge overhead movable light, a closet full of strange looking medical supplies and getting sicker by the minute. I had a flu-like nausea accompanied by severe diarrhea that had now turned to blood.

Needless to say, I made it through the first 24 hours and was about to embark on my first weeklong encounter with modern medicine.

Chapter 2

Week One - So what is This Thing?

After the emergency room experience, I woke up in a strange, dark room surrounded by my wife, two of our three daughters (one from North Carolina and the other from our hometown of Syracuse) and Jeff the Elder*.

Jeff informed me I was lucky to be alive and he would need to run a number of tests to see if any permanent damage had occurred. For the first time, MRI, CT scan and EKG became more than just vague medical terms to me. They looked for damage to the brain, heart and other organs.

According to a neurologist who stopped in later in the day, I had suffered a slight hemorrhage in my brain but it apparently did no permanent damage and should heal by itself. I would experience some fairly severe headaches for a few days but otherwise everything regarding my head and brain should return to normal.

During his rounds on Tuesday evening Jeff advised us that Myelodysplasia Refractory Anemia or MDS/RA was the tentative diagnosis. Remembering his comment about hoping for Leukemia, I asked what this new diagnosis was all about.

He was straightforward in telling me that MDS - my initial diagnosis and Aplastic Anemia (Myelodysplasia, Aplastic Anemia and a third disease called Paroxysmal Nocturnal Hemoglobinuria are easily confused in the laboratory and it is often necessary to have several biopsies performed to make the ultimate determination of which disease is present - since they are very closely related and the treatment protocol is the same, it really doesn't much matter what they are called) were serious, chronic diseases that were eventually fatal and I needed to "get my affairs in order".

*Dr. Jeffrey Kirshner of Hematology Oncology Associates of Central New York and the oldest of my three doctors named Jeff.

There it was - harsh reality and I could tell by the looks on the faces of the loved ones around me that this was not going to be a walk in the park. We were talking about being at death's door here and I needed to brace myself for the battle of my life.

Was this thing called MDS or its cousin AA an inherited condition?

This and other questions were asked while the PRBC's were being delivered intravenously to my blood starved body.

The Elder again assured me that Dad's Hodgkin's and my condition were not related. This man who recently saved my life was becoming a trusted confidant. He told me that MDS and AA are considered to be "idiopathic" - another term for my quickly growing medical dictionary.

In layman's terms, idiopathic means, "we don't really know." Accustomed to being able to ascertain anything about anything, I am not at all comfortable with such a definition when it was my life that was on the line. The term dysplasia refers to cells being of an abnormal size, development or structure and is often a precursor to cancer.

Severe Aplastic Anemia can, especially if untreated, advance to acute myelogenous leukemia, but also erythroleukemia and acute myelomonocytic leukemia in a relatively small number of cases (less than 15%). These are all very serious forms of leukemia, but they are treatable.

I began reading about the potential causes of aplastic anemia and found a great deal of speculation but very few facts. Benzene has been linked AA, MDS and Leukemia. Others believe that many medications or toxic substances in our environment may be to blame, but the conventional wisdom is that the cause is idiopathic.

Aplastic anemia is caused by bone marrow failure, resulting in poorly developed blood cells. Because the cells are malformed, they are destroyed by the patient's own immune system. There is a much more thorough discussion of the illness in the chapter called Aplastic Anemia Defined.

Severe aplastic anemia typically has a poor prognosis and can progress to leukemia, whereas pancytopenia may be reversible. Benzene-induced aplastic anemia is generally caused by chronic exposure at relatively high doses.

Fatal aplastic anemia following benzene exposure was first reported in workers in the nineteenth century but according to the NIH, that risk has been severely curtailed and the causes behind most current cases is unclear.

Wednesday evening, Sue and Melissa finally went home to get some much-deserved rest. Fred and Melanie had arrived from North Carolina and offered to camp out on my hospital room floor. Fred curled up on the floor in a blanket delivered by a helpful nurse and Melanie occupied the recliner. I don't know where all the hospitals get those recliners, but every one of them has a board right where your back wants to be – comfortable they are not!

* * * * *

"Momma called the doctor, momma called the nurse, momma called the lady with the alligator purse - In came the doctor, in came the nurse in came the lady with alligator purse - bad news said the doctor, bad news said the nurse, bad news said the lady with the alligator purse!"

Suddenly, my story as a patient in Community General Hospital had taken another dramatic turn. While recovering in my little private suite, I began shaking uncontrollably, rousing Fred and Melanie from their makeshift beds on the floor and in the recliner.

I was experiencing full body convulsions. I don't remember many of the details but just when I thought I was out of the woods, my whole body was shaking uncontrollably and my head felt like it was about to explode.

Somehow they calmed me down, gave me some kind of medication and I was told to rest while they paged the neurosurgeon on call. Oh great, I thought, what next? What was wrong with me? The neurologist on call showed up and after checking me out, ordered a CT scan and an MRI. Later results proved negative and he suggested the episode was probably just left over trauma from the entire experience.

Sue and Melissa had been summoned to my bedside for the third time in less than twenty-four hours - They had gone home hoping to catch some rest for the first time in two days. The stress on family members during these initial stages is incredible! Melanie tells me (I have only vague recollections) that I cried like a baby in her arms and said I did not want to die.

The next week became one of the most disconcerting weeks of my life. Remaining in the hospital because of my weakened position, the Elder informed me that I had experienced "a bleed to the brain, or a sub dermal hematoma".

They poked me and prodded every part of my body checking to see if anything else had been damaged during the remainder of my first one-week stay at CGH. Meanwhile my "counts" finally stabilized enough to send me home and await the next chapter in this new life.

I then settled in for regular visits to Hematology and Oncology Associates of Central New York (HOACNY) to check my blood counts usually followed by trips to the Community General Hospital's "Home Tonight" department for transfusions of the vital platelets and Packed Red Blood Cells or PRBC's needed to carry oxygen.

My buddy Jack, Wife Sue, Daughters and Sons-In Law, God-daughter Danielle, her mom, Dottie and many others later become platelet and blood donors.

The normal platelet transfusion process takes about thirty minutes but because I suffered allergic reactions early on, mine transfusions always took at least two hours each and if I needed both PRBC's and platelets, it was an all-day event. But I was alive and now consumed with trying to figure out what had gone wrong with my life.

Note - After several minutes of frantically searching around the hospital during Melanie's crisis, I located Adam and his mother. He suffered some minor cuts and bruises and had been unconscious when the ambulance arrived but he and Melanie fully recovered from their early brush with death.

Chapter 3

From the Beginning

A Brief Biography

This was not the first time I had been seriously ill. Family stories report that I battled for my life as a newborn, during the original baby boom.

My mother, Margaret Malina Nelson Lande delivered her bouncing baby boy on "one of the hottest August days anyone could remember." They tell me that Meningitis was the culprit and that I almost died at the tender young age of six months.

For the record, the birth occurred in one of the small almost nameless towns in northern Iowa or southern Minnesota or eastern South Dakota where my parents chased the dream of becoming full-fledged middle class citizens along with most of the WWII vets at the time. My dad managed a grain elevator like his father before him and the date was August 23, 1948.

My grandfather "Papa" as he was known to all eight of the Lande siblings, and my Grandmother Emma Lande raised a close-knit family that returned to the homestead in Elk Point, South Dakota every Christmas and again for an annual summer reunion. Twenty-three cousins fondly remember the times in Grandma's attic or the occasion of our graduation from the kids' table in the kitchen to the big people's holiday table in the huge dining room.

The elevator manager in a small town was akin to the bank manager or the mayor since nearly the entire populace relied on farming in one fashion or another in those days following the war. Rows of little houses were popping up everywhere and the family farm flourished feeding all the new arrivals during the post war baby boom.

Many of the farmers would mumble "munga tousen tak"* or a similar unintelligible phrase after my father unloaded their grain trucks. We are told that smell can spark memories better than any of the senses. The musty smell of dry grain brings me back to the wood covered floor of my Dad's little empire. Less than three or four years old, it is one of my first childhood memories.

That smell was again a part of my life while as a teen working on Farmer Brown's (that was his real name), homestead a few miles outside of Appleton, Minnesota, my hometown during the formative teen-age years. One of our jobs as "hired hands" was to drag corn down from the "cribs" using long corn rakes to ready the cobs for shelling.

The dried ears of corn would eventually be the primary ingredients fed to the award winning Angus Beef Cattle so prevalent in my boyhood version of Fargo. "Ya, sure you betcha!" That summer was one of the first times I remember suffering any kind of allergic reaction. I would come home from baling hay or pulling corn and have to soak in a tub full of water and baking soda to relieve the hives and itching sensation on my skin.

* * * * *

As my Dad told his story, he was approached by a recruiter for a large national company and urged to begin a new career selling crop hail insurance. He was eventually lured away from his esteemed position as WWII veteran and grain elevator manager in Larchwood, Iowa somewhere around 1951 or 1952.

Before you could say Fargo, North Dakota with a straight face, we were on our way to another small town in search of the American dream complete with a two-story house, two cars in the garage and golf at the local country club.

We settled in Willmar, Minnesota for about six years where he became the premier State Farm Insurance agent and, according to family legend, built the business into one of the largest auto, life, and health agencies in the state. He was developing a strong reputation both in our small town and the industry. He was well on his way to making a name for himself in what sister Martha thinks of as her hometown. Then, from out of nowhere, the two-car garage and dreams of a Horatio Alger story got hit with the first of many sucker punches.

Then in his early thirties and a prominent member of the local Jaycee's, Maynard Marion Lande, known to his friends and family as Maynard (who would name their son Marion - or Maynard for that matter?) was diagnosed with Hodgkin's disease.

Hodgkin's is another often-fatal disease of the Lymphatic system that, in my mind, sounded very similar to the diagnosis that had been explained to me by Dr. Kirshner.

* This means "many thousand thanks" and is the only phrase I know in my grandparent's native Norwegian tongue.

* * * * *

As for me, I played competitive basketball into my late 40's, still played golf to an 8 handicap in my early 50's and bounded upstairs two at a time. Suddenly, it was an effort to get out of a chair! It was like a permanent flu that would just not go away. Just the previous summer, my youngest daughter and I challenged my middle daughter and her husband to a basketball game and we whooped 'em bad! (OK, so we only played to five because I get winded after that but it was my court and my rules and Melanie and Fred claim it was Melissa and I left lying on the ground defeated.)

All three of our daughters had by then graduated from college and Sue and I were settling in to enjoy the beginning of our pre-retirement golden years.

We had recently moved into a new and larger (go figure) house in a really nice area with a swimming pool and were throwing parties like there was no tomorrow (little did we know at the time). In our own version of the "rags to riches" story, we thought we were on our way. Little did we know we were about to be rendered our own sucker punch!

Sue is a school nurse and I was the president, sales vice president, and head janitor for a burgeoning web site development business that had outgrown the basement of our old house - hence the move into a bigger house. With the smell of success in the air, we were hiring people and latching on to the technology boom. We were expanding into North Carolina in hopes of eventually moving the company headquarters to a warmer climate.

The large basement of our new house was renovated and dedicated to "hosting" the business. We had ten employees in two states that counted on us for their livelihood and then - the roof fell in!

Author's note – Several sections of the book contain entries from my personal journal. All entries have been edited, but some were left in their original form to better reflect the mood swings, alternating between elation and despair, great hope for the future and wondering if there would be another day.

Chapter 4

The Weakness Increases

June, 2000 – January, 2001

As alluded to in previous chapters, I officially grew up in rural Minnesota - actually went to college in "Fargo" but now lived in Syracuse, New York - the natives are quick to point out that Syracuse is in "Upstate" and therefore not to be confused with "The City." It really is a beautiful part of the country in the summer time, but like my native Minnesota, you can have it from December to March.

But in the summer time, I walked eighteen holes of golf on a regular basis and was the picture of health. This all began to change early in 2000 and I made my first visit to a doctor in over ten years. After much cajoling from Sue, I finally made an appointment to see my General Practitioner for a physical in July.

He did not find anything seriously wrong at that time and urged me to accept the fact that I was no longer a teenager and just needed to "slow down a bit". I went back to work at building our fledgling computer services and website development company with the same vigor as before.

My personal motto had always been to live each day with gusto and be in constant search of new challenges. I was not really one to take extreme physical risks ala skydiving or dirt biking, but I did enjoy the risks and rewards of taking on something new.

My most recent adventure had been to start an old time rock and roll band, ala CCR (Credence Clearwater Revival.) Our best "gig" was playing the Inauguration Ball for the Mayor of Rome (New York, not Italy). We also played a two-day overnighter for a biker wedding. What a blast! I prided myself on being a quick study and would take on new challenges with a zest that sometimes frustrated Sue.

As a kid growing up in the sixties, you had two choices - either start a garage band or join the football team. I opted for the latter, but always harbored a secret desire for the former. Whilst the young musicians were learning their riffs in the garage, I was being battered around on the gridiron. As the tallest, slowest, lightest member of the team, I held my own and even earned all-conference honors in my senior year.

I was also a pretty fair hoops player and spent my summers on the school links team long before golf was a "real" sport. Before Tiger blessed the now popular sport with his athletic prowess we golfers were considered wimps. Sue thinks that the predominant cause of my Aplastic Anemia stems from my habit of chewing on bits of clover and popping the golf ball in my mouth for cleaning prior to sinking a much needed birdie putt*. Herbicides and pesticides are listed as probable causes for Aplastic Anemia. I wonder if my boyhood idol, Arnold Palmer ever cleaned his golf ball that way.

So when my first official midlife crisis appeared in my early forties, starting an Eagles style garage band seemed highly logical. Our "sound" was intended to be a blend of early Buddy Holly and later Credence Clearwater Revival. Unfortunately our only "revival" efforts would be trying to rouse the bar stool occupants in a few of the remaining nightspots in the Salt City's dwindling nightlife.

What we lacked in musical harmony, we more than made up for in volume. Sue would claim she could hear the bass drum from two blocks away and our very own "groupies" constantly suggested we "turn it down!" It is fair to say that one of our members was actually an accomplished musician.

Early on, I wandered into a local guitar shop and after introducing myself to the manager, inquired about any local bands that might be in search of an average guitar player, come late blooming musician. The eventual "front man" for the "Reflections Two" responded that he would be interested in helping get a group like that off the ground. "You guys get your starts and stops down and come back to see me," said my newfound hero of the hop.

"I practiced all day and up into the night, my papa's hair was a turnin' white, cause he didn't like that rock and roll, he said you can stay son, but that's gotta go." -- Bobby Bare

After several months, Johnny agreed we were ready for prime time and joined our fledgling group. After another few months of less than successful outings he finally gave up on us and moved on to bigger and better things. Alas, my short-lived career as "The Boss" had come to an end. The only thing I had in common with Mr. Springsteen was our given names and a permanent ringing in my ears. My first midlife crisis had come to an end.

In addition to providing the color our band needed, Johnny also kept us entertained with his stories of the road. He claims to have fronted for The Boss and the E street band and later when he ran into Bruce in a local haunt, asked him stop by his table and say hello to impress his girlfriend.

The Boss says,

"Sure, happy to oblige."

Then dutifully stops by saying,

"Johnny, how ya doin' man, it's been a long time."

To which Johnny replies with a straight face,

"Not now, Bruce, can't you see I'm busy here."

* * * * *

About ten days prior to my visit to the Emergency Room, I pulled an all-nighter getting a customer's new computer system ready for them to start business the next day. I trudged up and down a twenty-step flight of stairs lugging heavy boxes. Sure, I grabbed the wall a couple of times, but just attributed it to working too hard. That night I had the mini-stoke that resulted in the bleed to the brain.

Being of strong Scandinavian stock, I got up and "walked it off." It wasn't until my Sister in Law, Gayle said "You look terrible, why are you so yellow?" during the Christmas celebration at our house that I began to appreciate something might be seriously wrong. Gayle doesn't usually pull any punches, but her frankness on this occasion took me by surprise.

Sue had been concerned for a long time about my jaundice color and the unexplained bruising, but I was too busy to take her seriously. I promised her I would rest up and not return to working my sixteen-hour days until after the holidays.

After Gayle's comment and more urging from Sue and my daughters, I finally relented to their constant pleas to return to the doctor for another checkup.

So early Monday morning, January 8, 2001 after a few preliminary tests by a nurse I made a return visit to what we used to call the Family Doctor and we now refer to as a General Practitioner. He took one look at me and spoke the words I will likely remember for the rest of my life,

"Something is seriously wrong, we don't know what it is yet, but look at your hand next to mine."

He rolled his palm up next to mine and I finally saw what everyone had been talking about. His palm was a healthy pink and mine was an ugly, grayish yellow.

Sue had been asking me for some time to explain the abnormal bruises and little read spots around my body and encouraging me to go to the doctor. I attributed the bruises to lugging the boxes and banging around in my normal haphazard style.

In my earlier days, I physically built two houses and still did lots of odd jobs around the house subjecting my body to all kinds of abnormal positions and tortures so bruises were pretty normal. The little red spots (later diagnosed as a petechial hemorrhage) were not as easily explained but "they would go away with time."

She had also advised me that I was cyanotic (the tips of my finger nails were pale blue rather than rosy pink) but I laughed that one off also. Sue knew something was wrong and had been urging me to see the doctor again for quite a while.

I was too busy with getting the new business off the ground and couldn't stop. Prior to the launching of the website development business, nearly all of my adult life had been spent in the computer business primarily in sales and sales management. I had a four-year college degree in Business Management and had always been a good provider if not an excellent father.

Sure, I loved our daughters but was more focused on building my career and chasing after my own version of Horatio Alger's story and living out my Renaissance man scenario while they were growing up.

Michelle inherited my passion for my music. She is an elementary teacher and self-taught musician. She had not had an easy life but through it all had somehow managed to not only graduate from high school, but also go on to college and earn her degree in elementary education.

Melanie got my athleticism. She was an award-winning gymnast before growing too tall for the sport. She cursed my 6'3" at the time but has grown to appreciate her strikingly good looks (from her Mother) and height from me.

Melissa inherited my passion for business. She kept the business alive and now runs it by herself. She also taught herself to play the drums so we could jam and learned to play basketball to spend more time with her Dad. She was the smart one-- Hmm, want Dad's attention; find a way to do what he loves. Now she is taking up golf.

* * * * *

By the time the Christmas holidays arrived I was pretty much unable to go up three steps without grabbing a wall for support. Gayle and others commented on how pale I looked, I had strange bruises and Sue again urged me to go see the Doctor. I visited Dr. Jeff Carlberg (Jeff the First) for the second time on January 8th.

After drawing some blood and running a few tests, the First did his "compare your hand to mine" bit and officially declared me a "very sick man". He arranged for me to see a Hematologist/Oncologist the next day and sent me home to wonder what was happening.

A Hematologist/Oncologist - what's that I wonder to myself? Blood and cancer I decide. Hmmm - this does not sound good. Early the next day, the Hematologist's office called advising me to get the Emergency Room as quickly as possible. Oh-oh must be something seriously wrong. I had been expecting a routine visit to his office.

I then began experiencing the efficiencies and unfortunately many of the deficiencies of our modern medical system. Evidently Jeff the Elder's office had called ahead and they were actually expecting me at the Emergency Room that is only a few minutes from our new home. Before I could even comprehend what was happening, I was lying on a gurney (that skinny little thing that is way too short for my 6'3" height) in the ER with Sue and Melissa standing guard.

I thank God daily for my wife and her experience as a Registered Nurse. I am convinced neither me nor my Father in Law would still be on this earth if not for the prompt action and dogged bedside assistance rendered by her and her sister Kathie. They both know how things can go wrong and were not going to let it happen to me!

Now that you have a sense of the initial hospital experience and my life prior to January of 2001, it's time to get "grounded" on the illnesses and the conventional ways of dealing with them.

Chapter 5

Aplastic Anemia Defined

AA, MDS and the Others

According to the Aplastic and MDS International Foundation, Inc.:

"Aplastic Anemia and Myelodysplastic Syndromes can strike any person of any age, of any gender or any race, of any neighborhood anywhere in the world. In the United States, thousands of men, women and children are stricken with these non-contagious and often fatal blood disorders every year. They occur when the bone marrow stops making enough healthy blood cells. In most cases the cause of the diseases is idiopathic (unknown.) The suspected causes are many: radiation, benzene-based compounds, viruses such as hepatitis; environmental toxins; over the counter and prescription medications; street drugs; and other many chemicals too numerous to list."

One of the first noticeable symptoms of Aplastic Anemia is petechiae in your eyes or elsewhere. Another symptom that should have been like a fire alarm but I ignored was constant blood in my nose and mouth. You may also see bruises on different parts of your body with no recollection of what may have caused them.

If you encounter these symptoms, there is very likely something seriously wrong with you. Call your doctor and/or get yourself to the emergency room ASAP! You are bleeding internally and need medical attention NOW! My first trip to the ER, my platelet count was 3,000 vs. a normal 100,000 - 300,000. I did not have enough platelets to stop the internal bleeding.

According to the Rush Cancer Center in Chicago,

"Aplastic anemia is a rare disease that strikes the bone marrow and produces a deficiency of red blood cells, white blood cells and platelets. Hemorrhages and other life- threatening disorders may accompany aplastic anemia; a bone marrow transplant is the only current effective treatment. Aplastic anemia patients who do not receive a bone marrow transplant may go on to develop myelodysplasia which, in turn, can progress to leukemia."

The official strategy for the treatment for Aplastic Anemia as espoused by the National Institute of Health goes as described below by Dr. Neil S. Young, the recognized authority on this illness in the United States.

Note: If you get lost in the middle, you may want to skip over the treatment strategy for now. It has taken me a long time to understand and I will explain it in more detail in the chapter on research.

"Immunosuppression is employed in patients who are not candidates for stem cell transplantation due either age or the lack of a donor. Antithymocyte Globulin (ATG), which is licensed for use in the United States, is a horse immunoglobulin preparation derived from the sera of animals immunized with normal pediatric thymus tissue. Hematologic responses, which are usually equivalent to sufficiently improved blood counts such that the patient no longer requires transfusions of red blood cells or platelets and is not susceptible to infection, occur in 40%-50% of those treated with either ATG or comparable European antilymphocyte globulins (ALG) . For patients with severe aplastic anemia, the addition of Cyclosporine to ATG or ALG has improved response and survival rates. In European and American studies, response rates have been 70%-80% and survival at 5 years among responders is about 90%. Combined treatment with Cyclosporine and ATG has been particularly beneficial for children and patients with absolute neutropenia compared with results for ATG alone. Cyclosporine as a single agent of immunosuppression is inferior to ATG or ALG.

ATG and ALG have distinctive toxicities. As foreign proteins, they can elicit anaphylaxis (A system or treatment that leads to damaging effects on the organism) in the host; we routinely skin test for evidence of sensitivity and desensitize patients who have a positive reaction. ATG is not specific for lymphocytes and can reduce already low platelet and neutrophil levels and convert the direct antiglobulin test. Antihorse antibodies produced by the patient can lead to immune complex formation and serum sickness, usually about 11 days after initiation of treatment .40 Cyclosporine is nephrotoxic and both serum creatinine and drug levels should be monitored to avoid irreversible renal damage. Hypertension, gingival hyperplasia, and gastrointestinal and neurologic symptoms are other common side effects. Because of the risk of Pneumocystis carinii, we administer prophylaxis with monthly pentamidine inhalations.

Many (perhaps most) patients with aplastic anemia are not adequately treated by a single 4-day course of ATG followed by 6 to 12 months of Cyclosporine. Slowly declining blood counts signal a need to retreat and usually respond to either an increase in the dose or the reinstitution of Cyclosporine. Some patients appear to depend on continued administration of Cyclosporine, often at relatively low doses. Less frequently, as in the current case, frank pancytopenia recurs and requires a second course of ATG.

However, long-term prognosis does not appear to be affected by relapse. Patients who respond to immunosuppression often continue to have blood counts that, while adequate for full activities, remain below normal. Incomplete responses, frequent relapses, and Cyclosporine dependence are probably evidence of chronic immune system activity in a hematologically compensated bone marrow.

Only a few patients face an actual choice between allogenic transplantation and immunosuppressive therapy. Analyses of large databases have not shown major differences in outcomes between these two therapeutic approaches. Nevertheless, transplant is probably preferable for certain defined subgroups, especially young patients and those with very severe neutropenia. Patients who failed immunosuppressive therapy have later undergone successful transplantation from matched siblings or from unrelated donors.

ATG and ALG reduce lymphocyte numbers, but transiently and modestly compared with cytotoxic chemotherapy; part of their beneficial activity may be to induce tolerance, perhaps by specific deletion of activated lymphocytes. Both these quantitative and qualitative mechanisms of action suggest alternative approaches to immunosuppression. Small numbers of patients reported to have responded to cyclophosphamide administered at high doses equivalent to those employed in transplant conditioning regimens but without stem cell rescue.

High dose cyclophosphamide is a much more aggressive form of immunosuppression than antilymphocyte sera and results in profound and sustained suppression of bone marrow function as well, but cyclophosphamide may have the advantage of inducing more complete hematologic responses, avoiding relapse, and preventing the development of late clonal diseases (see below). High-dose cyclophosphamide is compared with conventional ATG treatment in our current NIH randomized, crossover design protocol for patients with severe aplastic anemia.

Conversely, milder but more specific forms of immunosuppression might also be effective. For example, ATG contains antibody specificities for the interleukin-2 receptor, present on activated lymphocytes; we are testing a commercially available monoclonal antibody to the receptor in patients with moderate aplastic anemia. For prolonged immunosuppression, new oral agents like mycophenolate mofetil, which seems to induce tolerance and lacks Cyclosporine's nephrotoxicity, deserve testing as an addition to initial immunosuppressive regimens and at the time of relapse."

I read these definitions and treatment protocols over and over again trying to make sense of what was happening. I have always attempted to simplify things rather than allow them to become overcomplicated, but this was obviously not going to be an easy effort when nearly every other word was unfamiliar to me.

I was beginning to realize that since such a small number of people were diagnosed with Aplastic Anemia or Myelodysplastic Syndromes each year, this was not a set of illnesses that was receiving a whole lot of attention in the medical research community. My business head told me that small numbers meant limited funding and limited funding meant little hope for any miraculous discoveries that may suddenly come to my rescue. No, Bubba, you were going to be on your own this time!

We spent a considerable amount of time investigating the clinical trials that were in process. If you want to know what clinical trials are being conducted for your illness, go to http://www.centerwatch.com or one of the many other websites that track the trials.

According to the NIH, a clinical trial is a research study to answer specific questions about vaccines, new therapies or new ways of using known treatments. Clinical trials (also called medical research and research studies) are used to determine whether new drugs or treatments are both safe and effective. Carefully conducted clinical trials are the fastest and safest way to find treatments that work in people.

Participants in clinical trials can play a more active role in their own health care, gain access to new research treatments before they are widely available, and help others by contributing to medical research.

Ideas for clinical trials usually come from researchers. After researchers test new therapies or procedures in the laboratory and in animal studies, the treatments with the most promising laboratory results are moved into clinical trials. During a trial, more and more information is gained about a new treatment, its risks and how well it may or may not work.

Clinical trials are conducted in phases. The trials at each phase have a different purpose and help scientists answer different questions:

In Phase I trials, researchers test a new drug or treatment in a small group of people (20-80) for the first time to evaluate its safety, determine a safe dosage range, and identify side effects.

In Phase II trials, the study drug or treatment is given to a larger group of people (100-300) to see if it is effective and to further evaluate its safety.

In Phase III trials, the study drug or treatment is given to large groups of people (1,000-3,000) to confirm its effectiveness, monitor side effects, compare it to commonly used treatments, and collect information that will allow the drug or treatment to be used safely.

In Phase IV trials, post marketing studies delineate additional information including the drug's risks, benefits, and optimal use.

Over the years, there have been many treatment protocols that have been tried including bloodletting (actually this is still a common practice used to aid in the removal of iron – officially it is called phlebotomy), herbal treatments, Bone Marrow or Stem Cell Transplants and the most current strategy designed to suppress the immune system using various serums from animals (ATG from horse and ALG from Rabbit).

Here are all the protocols and treatments I have uncovered during my research to date:

Bone Marrow or Stem Cell Transplants

A Full Bone Marrow Transplant

There are several different types of full bone marrow transplants. The first level of differentiation is whether or not the patient's own marrow is used (autologous) or the marrow of someone else is used (allogenic).

The allogenic transplant may be provided by an HLA matched sibling or from a Matched Unrelated Donor (MUD).

There is an excellent description of the procedure at http://www.rushcancer.org/bmt/vabmt/vabmt.html.

Here is a synopsis:

There are generally three steps to an autologous (use of patient's own retreated marrow) bone marrow transplant.

1)   The first is receiving chemotherapy to reduce any cancer cells in the body to a minimum.

2)   The second is collection and storage of bone marrow cells.

3)   The third is the transplant itself. This involves giving high doses of chemotherapy with or without radiation, reinfusing the stem cells then waiting for the bone marrow function to return.

The following description is from the National Bone Marrow Center Web Page at http://www.marrow.org:

Early Stem Cell History

Nearly a century ago, physicians administered bone marrow by mouth to patients with anemia and leukemia. Although such therapy was unsuccessful, laboratory experimenters eventually demonstrated that mice with defective marrow could be restored to health with infusions into the blood stream of marrow taken from other mice.

This caused physicians to speculate whether it was feasible to transplant bone marrow from one human to another (allogenic transplantation). Among the early attempts to do this were several transplants carried out in France following a radiation accident in the late 1950's.

In a Full Bone Marrow Transplant, the patient or recipients bone marrow is completely destroyed using high dose chemotherapy. The donor's marrow is then infused into the recipient's body. The theory is that the donor's marrow will then function to regenerate healthy cells.

This procedure relies heavily on matching the HLA characteristics of the recipient and donor. The best possible match is from a twin, followed by and HLA matched sibling and finally by an unrelated donor. Because children of a recipient have HLA characteristics from both parents, it is virtually impossible that the child would match the parent and the opposite is also true.

The HLA System

The human leukocyte antigens or HLA antigens are proteins found on the surface of most cells in the body. These HLA antigens give the body's immune system the ability to determine what belongs in the body and what does not belong. Whenever the immune system does not recognize the series of antigens on a cell that mark it as belonging in the body, it creates antibodies and other substances to destroy the cell.

Objects that the body looks for and destroys are infection-causing bacteria, viruses, tumor cells and foreign objects such as splinters. In this way, the immune system defends the body against things that can enter the body and cause harm.

For a bone marrow transplant to work, the recipient's immune system must not try to destroy the donated marrow. This is accomplished by making sure that the antigens on the donated marrow cells are identical, or very similar to, the antigens on the cells of the recipient.

Each transplant center uses slightly different protocols, but the fundamental strategy is to weaken the immune system using Cyclosporine and/or a drug called Methotrexate and the patient is given multiple prophylactic drugs to minimize the effects of GVHD.

Once the immune system is weakened, then the bone marrow is destroyed using chemotherapy and finally the donor marrow is administered. The actual delivery of the marrow is pretty much a non-event. Less than one liter is delivered via IV over a relatively short period of time. By far the most critical issue is guarding against and treating the various symptoms associated with the GVHD.

My research has indicated that full bone marrow transplants are fully successful about 50% of the time. The primary complication in a bone marrow transplant is a phenomenon known as Graft vs. Host Disease or GVHD. With GVHD, the newly transplanted T-lymphocyte cells (a type of white blood cell responsible for destroying "non-self" invaders) of the donor recognizes the patients cells as being foreign and begins destroying the healthy cells.

There are two types of GVHD. The first is called Acute GVHD and it usually occurs within the first three months after the transplant. The second type is called chronic GVHD and it occurs later but persists for a longer time period.

In Acute GVHD, the T-Cells attack the patient's skin, liver, stomach, and/or intestines. The first signs of acute Graft-versus-Host disease are a skin rash that appears on the hand, feet, and face that may also spread to other parts of the body. The patient may also experience diarrhea and stomach cramps.

Doctors have learned to administer prophylactic medication in an effort to avoid GVHD, but these medications do not always work and the acute GVHD can be fatal or cause permanent damage to the various organs affected.

The second type of GVHD is called Chronic GVHD and it usually occurs after the patient has been discharged and the procedure appears to have been successful. It can occur anywhere from three months to as much as a year after the initial transplant.

The causes of chronic Graft-versus-Host disease are not clear, but it also is thought to involve the T cell from the donor. Initial symptoms include severe skin rashes and hair loss. Once present, chronic GVHD may attack virtually any organ in the body. The immune system essentially begins to malfunction and does not react properly to infections or other problems.

Chronic GVHD is a very serious condition that can be life threatening and it affects nearly 50% of all patients who undergo the transplant.

Transplant with T-Cell Depletion

A relatively new strategy as of 2001 is a protocol called T-cell depletion. In this strategy, the lymphocytes that cause GVHD are removed from the T cells before the marrow is transferred to the recipient.

You can become a donor or read more about the National Bone Marrow Center at http://www.marrow.org or contact them at:

National Marrow Donor Program Suite 500

3001 Broadway Street Northeast Minneapolis, MN 55413-1753

Phone Numbers:

In the United States and Canada, call toll free:

General Information: (800) MARROW2 (1-800-627-7692)

The Office of Patient Advocacy (OPA): (888) 999-6743

Outside the United States:

General Information: (612) 627-8141

The Office of Patient Advocacy (OPA): (612) 627-8140

Mini Transplants

The Mini Transplant requires less strenuous pre-transplant conditioning regimens and may be suitable for a wider range of patients, especially patients over the age of 55.

Doctors refer to this as a non-myeloablative transplant because it does not completely destroy the patient's diseased marrow.

Patients receive lowered doses of chemotherapy drugs, typically about 50% of the "normal" dose.

Mini transplant patients have what is called mixed chimerism. This means blood and marrow cells from both the donor and recipient coexist within the recipient's body. Eventually, the goal is for most, if not all, of the recipient's blood and marrow cells to be of donor origin.

The Mini transplant is not available to all patients and as of 2002 it is still considered somewhat experimental. Because it is new, the success rate is not yet well documented.

The transplant centers are continually searching for better ways to combat GVHD, as it is the most serious variable in dealing with any of the transplant strategies.

Immunosuppression Drug Based Strategies:

The most popular strategy for immunosuppression therapy as of 2001 is the administration of a horse serum (ATG) or a rabbit serum (ALG) that is designed to weaken the immune system and its response to the poorly formed blood cells associated with AA or MDS. There are also a wide variety of additional strategies being tried with MDS depending on the type and severity of the case.

The centers have also tried many other drug therapies including Methylprednisolone, Fludarabine, Danazol, Cyclosporine and Cytoxan or Cyclophosphamide. Other patients have also told me they have been threatened with Arsenic (now that sounds pretty dangerous) and many other drugs too numerous to mention. The response to all of these strategies varies all over the place and can take many months before success is achieved if at all.

Preliminary data from Johns Hopkins suggests that high-dose cyclophosphamide may result in durable remissions in some patients with aplastic anemia, but a recent report suggests that rates of fungal infections may practically limit this approach, and its use as of 2001 was limited to clinical trials.

Mindy and several other members of the website have achieved success with this protocol.

Herbal Treatments and Others

From http://www.lef.org/protocols/prtcl-009a.shtml

"A specific natural therapy to restore healthy platelet production is 5 capsules a day of standardized shark liver oil, containing 200 mg of alkylglycerols per capsule. Studies have shown that shark liver oil can boost the production of blood platelets. Studies have also shown the immune enhancement capabilities of shark liver oil (J. Alt. Compl. Med., 1998 Spring; 4 [1]: 87-99). "

Melatonin has also been reported to be an especially effective and safe therapy to treat thrombocytopenia but I rather doubt it because it also claims to cure everything from athlete's foot to insomnia.

From a website member:

"My son was diagnosed with AA in Sept of 98. I have been reading everyone's report and have written a few times. He had ATG and was on cyclosporine for about a year and then refused to take it because it made him gag and he felt sick. He just quit taking it. The Dr. put him on Prograph and it was a lot better. He took it for about 3 months and at this point has quit taking it.

We have decided to go with alternative healing since the Dr's don't really know how to treat this dreadful disease. He started having auricular acupuncture and natural healing in Feb of this year.

He is taking a liquid supplement called sea silver, colostrum and shark liver oil great immune boosters and milk thistle and dong quai. His platelet count in Jan was 75,000 as of April they are 150.000.

Fish Oil – I do not recommend this one, but read on...

Fish oil has many names. One of the most common is omega-3 fatty acid or its scientific abbreviation, N-3. N3 fatty acids are found mostly in fish, but are contained in other foods as well. Fish oil is the best food source of these fatty acids.

The primary benefit of N-3 fish oil is the reduction of platelet activity (blood clotting) and plaque formation that in turn can prevent heart attacks. The nutritionist at EHCD had me on omega 3!

Here's how it works. Platelets are clot-forming blood cells that prevent excessive bleeding. Overly active platelets, however, may speed the build-up of plaque, a deposit of fatty or fibrous material that narrows a blood vessel wall. Elevated blood cholesterol also contributes to the acceleration of plaque formation. When plaque narrows an artery it is easier for a blood clot to get stuck in the artery and this can cause a heart attack. Because platelets also form blood clots, this is likely to occur. That's why it is desirable to reduce platelet activity and why N-3 fatty acid, fish oil, is beneficial.

From the ITP website:

Finally my only choices were chemotherapy or experimental procedures. My father started researching and found Dr. Ba. Although I've only spoken to him on the phone, he's helped me so much. He got me started on this tea called Radix Rehmanniae Preparata and some in a pill form. It's a cake like tea that doesn't taste that good.

After drinking two cups a day and four of the pills my platelets increased by 10,000 even after I started to wean myself off the prednisone. In May 1999 my platelets are at 70,000. My last prednisone was June2. Now on July 1999 I'm at 258,000. I still take my normal vitamins and now the Chinese pills. I really hate this illness but this was more like a blessing in disguise.... to take better care of myself.

Several members swear by Chinese medicines and doctors they have investigated. I was likely going to try that next had the regimen I am using did not work.

Caution – Most doctors advise against using herbal treatments in conjunction with drug therapies.

Alternative Treatments

The alternative treatments I use and recommend are thoroughly discussed in the chapter on holistic healing. There are many other alternative treatments that have been attempted by various members and that I have read about in cancer prevention books, books on nutrition, books by Dr. Rogers and many others.

The alternative treatments vary considerably and I have obviously not tested every one. There are, however several common themes that appear in most of the alternative therapies that have been discussed. They include, but are not necessarily limited to:

- Fresh, clean spring water
- At least an hour of sunshine each day
- At least sixty minutes of exercise each day
- No sugar, processed food and junk food
- No alcohol, tobacco, caffeine or soda of any kind

- Reducing or eliminating stress
- A means of achieving inner peace
- Healing and/or cleansing the gut
- Limiting the use of medications and drugs

Foods and supplements can often contradict as noted here:

- Eating only raw vegetables
- Eating only cooked vegetables
- Eating a diet high in protein including liver
- Barley green powder
- A cup of popcorn every day
- Sesame seeds and/or sesame oil
- A rotation diet
- Grains, greens and beans diet
- Macrobiotic diet
- Mega doses of virtually every vitamin & supplement

As you can see, there more ideas and alternative treatments available than any one person could try. I rejected many of the more outlandish ones immediately but did try to at least investigate the ones that seemed reasonable and tried a few with minimal results. There are many more alternative treatments discussed http://aplasticcentral.org and you can read about success stories in the member's section and the forum. The website is free to all users and is updated on a regular basis.

Symptoms and Issues

The following is a list of symptoms and issues that are directly related to AA or my stay in the hospital:

Caked blood in nose and blood in mouth in AM

Bruising – abnormally sized black, blue and yellow spots

Cyanotic – White fingernails –Compare yours to others
Yellow Palms – Ditto above
Neuropathy – Loss of feeling in feet due to poor circulation

Fatigue – Comes and goes and I try to rest when it comes
Unable to exert – Can't lift heavy objects or run or jump

Mood swings
A sharp tinge of pain occasionally at catheter site
Really dry skin at times

Severe muscle cramps in toes and shins
Arthritis like cramping and weakness in fingers

Many of the above symptoms are caused by poor circulation and the lack of oxygen being properly distributed throughout the body, especially extremities.

Speculation on Causes

I hint at possible causes throughout the book. Here is a summary of items that I think may have contributed listed in order of my suspicion:

Pesticides and Herbicides from golf ball and golf course

Varnishing in a closed basement 2-3 years before

Extensive dental work removing amalgam 1 year before

Spending far too much time in a very moldy basement
Radon in one of two houses we lived in
Chronic tonsillitis – see chapter on immune system

Chronic sinusitis – ditto above
Spreading and spraying stuff on lawn
Mega doses of Vitamin C

Daily Aspirin to ward off heart disease
Antibiotics for sore throats at least twice a year

Shingles – Herpes Zoster Virus
Working in a fertilizer plant as a teen
Meningitis as a child

Fast food junkie
A cleaning fluid used in an office building where I worked
I often siphoned gas by mouth until about 1985 (brilliant!)

Heavy smoker from 20's to 30's

I don't believe that any one thing caused my Aplastic Anemia but rather that it was a combination of many of the above issues and the continued abuse of my body over so many years.

I eventually decided that finding the cause was far less important than finding the cure, so my challenge is to see if I can reverse the process by taking better care of myself and adapting a holistic approach to life.

I have been using myself as a human test lab for about two years now trying everything that made sense and a few things that did not. Interestingly enough after all the research I have done, the ones that make the least sense to me are the conventional wisdom approaches of rabbit serum, horse serum and cyclosporine. They supposedly are working for others but the sound utterly bizarre to me.

My suspicion and as was pointed out by one of the aplastic central forum members is that "time" is one of the best medicines. We need to take better care of ourselves, take transfusions as necessary, but then rely on our body to eventually heal itself. In the meantime, I personally believe that we should avoid all the drugs typically prescribed and opt for a natural approach to healing.

To give you a sense of my ongoing research, as I write the book, I am reading the Prescription for Nutritional Healing and happened across a section on fasting that supposedly helps heal the immune system so I decided to give it a try. You can read about the process in the chapter on detoxing and nutrition.

Because every one of us is different with our own histories and bodies, it is important to read everything you can find and conduct your own research into what you may think will work for you. In the end, each one of us is responsible for our own decisions and our own health.

Please see the chapter on holistic medicine to see what regimen I follow and refer to the website for additional information on treatment strategies others have tried.

Chapter 6

Settling In for the Long Haul

Life As I Knew It Was Over

What had started out as another interesting adventure had now turned into a battle for my life. Not fully comprehending the serious nature of my illness until I was officially diagnosed as "non-responsive" to two rounds of therapeutic "ATG" treatments, I was fighting and losing in the battle to regain control of my everyday life. Every day seemed to find me weaker and caught in a devastating catch twenty-two.

My blood could not support exercise and the more days that went by without exercise the weaker I became.

Following are the journal entries as my "new life" began:

January 15, 2001

Released from CGH and was told to take it very easy and would be seeing Hematologist twice a week for CBC*. I was also advised to set up an appointment in Rochester for further testing and diagnosis. The original biopsy report was sent to Strong Memorial for their review.

My brother Greg and sister Martha were alerted as possible sibling donors for an anticipated bone marrow transplant. They quickly went to local clinics and we waited for results.

According to one of the attending physicians who shall remain nameless, if I had more than thirty Platelet Transfusions or twenty PRBC Transfusions I would likely die of complications.

We later learned this was incorrect, but it had us very upset for quite a while, as I had received six such transfusions in the month of January alone. We quickly calculated that I would not last past July at this rate.

I began charting my transfusions and diligently recorded each event in a spreadsheet. After about six months of this activity with nothing changing, I finally gave it up for more meaningful pursuits.

*CBC (Complete Blood Count) See complete definitions in the glossary.

* * * * *

Having survived that first frightening night, I began to ask the inevitable questions: Why me? How did this happen? What causes this type of illness? How long will I live? Is it contagious? Is it hereditary? Would my father's Hodgkin's have been lingering in my body all these years? What about my sister's Lupus? Are my kid's in danger? What can I do to fight this intruder?

The next setting in this challenging life adventure was a small, yet surprisingly comfortable private room in my wife's old digs. She knew most of the nurses from her days of "floating" to multiple floors while employed at Community General Hospital - sounds like a good name for a soap opera, doesn't it?

I later learn that she and her friends pulled a few strings to get me my privacy but then I am also informed that the isolation is critical since my resistance to disease is very low. Condition-wise, I am bordering on neutropenia - an extremely low White Blood Cell count. My personal dictionary is expanding faster than the Mississippi River during the spring thaw.

* * * * *

Mississippi was one of the first really complex words I learned to spell along with my fellow boomers sweating it out in Mrs. Anderson's second grade class. I was usually anxious to get on the playground to practice my new hook shot, but managed to pull good enough elementary school grades to be transferred to the new experimental gifted class by the time I reached sixth grade.

By that time, we had moved at least six different times and though I had burgeoning friendships in many small towns in the Midwest, I had not yet stayed in one place long enough to develop any strong relationships.

My Dad's battle with Hodgkin's had reached an impasse (after 12-18 months of sheer hell according to my sister and others), and he graciously volunteered to coach the Pee Wee basketball team where I achieved one of my first claims to fame. You could probably never find the records to prove me right (or wrong), but I was the leading scorer in the Willmar, Minnesota Pee Wee basketball program.

I was a mean driver of the lane ala Elgin Baylor and possessed a great Pistol Pete style "shoot from the hip" jump shot. I was not strong enough to get the ball into the appropriate position for shooting, so would launch from my hip like hoisting a bag of fertilizer to your shoulder. I learned this fine art during the summer of my senior year in high school (yes, in yet another small mid-western stop that became "my" hometown). It is here that I was exposed to another probable cause.

While taking a break from chasing all the eligible young blondes in our little hamlet of transplanted Norwegians and Swedes, I worked a summer job that required the daily inhalation of potassium dust, ammonia fumes and all sorts of other nasty smelling chemicals at the local Midland Co-Operative Fertilizer outlet.

I worked for a gentlemanly fellow by the unusual name of Floyd Wojtalewicz (I learned to spell his name so I could sign his name on receiving documents), the only Polish American our small mostly Scandinavian town ever knew. Little did I know that one of my closest friends and best golfing buddies was named Ray Stackowicz, and I would round out my spelling lessons with another weird sounding Polish name.

While my eventual wife was growing up in a more naturally fertilized world in Upstate New York (Not to be confused with Downstate where all the politicians come from), I was ingesting all sorts of foul smelling manmade derivatives that are probably still floating around in my body someplace. The more natural, organic fertilizer Sue grew up with was courtesy of the 60 or so horses owned by her father.

Next to my own Dad, her Dad and my Father-In-Law, Art, is the man I admire most. You will never see his name in "Who's Who of America," but in his own way, he made history in the Scenic Valley of Sue's youth. Together with my second mom Dorothy "Dot" Burghardt, Art was the proprietor of the Scenic Valley Riding Stables for over forty years. While my family was moving from one small mid-western town to another, Art and Dottie stayed put in the little country farmhouse where they still live today.

Together, they nurtured horses and kids and spread more love than any couple I have ever met. The "Riding Stables" has been closed since the 90's but they still receive Christmas Cards from all over the country. Here's one I read last week from the Southeastern U.S.: "Art, do you remember me? You used to make me ride Admiral and would always kid me that he would buck me off. Well he never did and I now have an Admiral of my own here on my little horse farm in Virginia. Hope to see you when we come to Syracuse this summer. Love, Laurie"

Or this card from North of the Border: "Dot - I remember when you started our 4-H group and you spent so many hours with me chasing the horses into the barn, cleaning them up and then cooking one of your special open fire dinners for us. I now live in Canada and have my own horse. Love, Cheryl."

Their kitchen walls are literally filled with these cards and pictures of the many kids they helped keep off the streets. Dot was also the resident nurse for a summer camp nearby when she wasn't working her full time job as a Registered Nurse. Art tended the horses while providing his Upstate New York version of Will Rogers' humor for the kids and their parents.

They hosted weekend trail rides in their beautiful valley nestled amongst the foothills of the Adirondack Mountains. They looked like mountains to my "so flat you can see all the way to Fargo" eyes, but Sue assured me they were only foothills and later took me for a tour of the real mountains of Northern New York.

Art was also quite the "horse trader" in his day and accumulated a barn full of antiques to go with his garage full of surreys and his clubroom full of wall hangings and tack room full of old saddles and stirrups from the civil war. The old homestead looks a lot like a shooting location for Sanford and Son, but the love and good times were abundant.

Following her cross country visit to meet my new-found love, my mother would remark at the number hungry cowboys that would saddle up to the table for "lunch." In between trail rides, the trail bosses would show up in the old country kitchen hungry for chicken and one of Arts' stories. On average, Dot served up twenty-five to thirty dinner sized lunches every weekend day all summer long for about twenty years.

The food was wholesome, the fertilizer was deep and organic and the impression on many others and me would last a lifetime.

* * * * *

According to my limited amount of scientific research, many of the chemicals associated with inorganic fertilizers can lay dormant in your body tissues for years similar to the nicotine deposits in your lungs that can reach up and grab you years after you have given up the ugly habit.

Succumbing to peer pressure, I took up the nasty habit early and did not give it up until just before Melissa; our youngest was born in 1976. My personal opinion is that this early habit was likely more of a cause than the aforementioned habit of popping fertilizer laden golf balls in my mouth for cleaning. Besides, who wants to believe that one's favorite pastime could be the cause of his eventual demise?

Did any of these cause my Aplastic Anemia? Was it smoking three packs of mostly filtered death sticks for over 15 years, chemicals from the fertilizer plant or fertilizer covered golf balls? Or maybe it was my bout with what a social worker termed "alcohol abuse? I had not had a single drink in over ten years, but the remnants of those early abuses were probably still resident in my liver and other places.

While lying on my back in a New York based community hospital fifteen hundred miles and twenty years away from my Minnesota youth I conjured up all sorts of suspected causes. The once precious commodity of "time to myself" was now in abundance and my mind raced around trying to make sense of my predicament.

Syracuse's Community General Hospital was once a proud statement to the prosperous and sprawling western suburbs, but had been slowly decaying over the past several years as the remains of Willis Carrier's Refrigerated Empire joined most other Northeastern Manufacturers in their flight south.

Once a bustling center of commerce on the ill-fated Erie Canal, the dwindling city is but one of the many cities you blow by on the New York State Thruway or Ohio Turnpike while traveling from Boston to Chicago. Gasoline and diesel fumes are also suspected causes of autoimmune related illnesses. As a result of my extensive reading, I have decided that Aplastic Anemia is but one version of a host of illnesses that can be directly related to our 21st century environment.

In the forward to Dr. Sherry Rogers book "Tired or Toxic," Dr. William Rea states: "This information is vitally important now as it touches everyone with nearly any symptom such as chemical sensitivity, high cholesterol, chronic fatigue, Candida-related complex, depression, Alzheimer's, high blood pressure, diabetes, heart disease, osteoporosis and more." As you will learn later, I credit these two modern day crusaders with nurturing me back to health.

Had it not been for these two doctors and Sue's constant, though gentle coercion, this book would not have been written and I would not be here to tell my story.

* * * * *

Chapter 7

Life According to Bubba

Setting the Stage

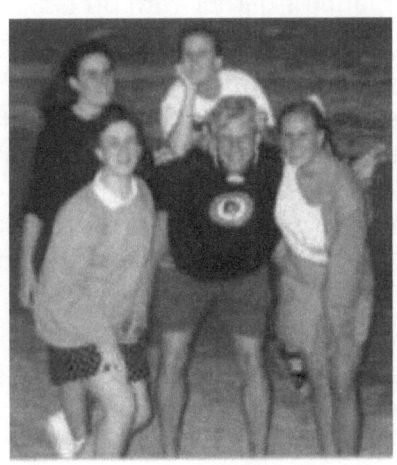

That's me in the middle of "My Girls" a few years before being diagnosed. The proud father of three girls and a loving wife of over thirty years, I was given six months to live in January of 2001. At times over the next few months I was not sure I even wanted to stick around given my quality of life at the time.

This book is a personal journal of my struggle with Aplastic Anemia and is a signpost for the many others of you who are encountering a life threatening illness for the first time. It is dedicated to my wife, family and friends in grateful appreciation for giving me the will to live and win my battle against AA.

Over the past two years, I have re-discovered my roots and set a new goal to find a lasting cure for Aplastic Anemia and similar Autoimmune Related Disorders and share the information I gather with others.

I have also chosen to tell my life story in hopes that it will help the reader understand that what is happening to me is something that can happen to anyone at any time. In our thirties we see the world as our oyster and think we are invincible. As we progress into later years, we realize how fragile life is on this earth and we appreciate each day God has given us.

"When the One Great Scorer comes to write against your name, He marks - not that you won or lost - but how you played the game", Grantland Rice.

* * * * *

A Message from Sue

Bruce is truly a remarkable man that I have had the pleasure of knowing and loving for the past 33 plus years. His knowledge and drive have never ceased to amaze me. (Sometimes his drive makes me crazy, but all in all, it is a big part of why I love him as I do.)

The world as we knew it came crashing down on us January 9th, 2001 with the diagnosis of Aplastic Anemia. I know that many of you have read his account, but now I will tell you mine. As the spouse of anyone with a life threatening illness, one somehow, if lucky, manages to get through the trying days - often an hour at a time. The love and support we received from our loved ones was what kept me going.

Our daughter Melissa kept our family business afloat so we could pay the mounting bills and buy some time to reconstruct our lives. She was a pillar of strength to me and to her Dad.

To her, I owe the deepest gratitude. To our other daughters, Melanie and Michelle and Sons-In Law, Mike and Fred, I also owe thanks from the bottom of my heart. Melanie and Michelle live in North Carolina and Florida so it was sometimes even harder for them being so far away at a time of family crisis.

They made several expensive trips home, offered whatever support they could and were a source of support to me when I needed them. Mike especially seemed to be there when I needed him - mowing the lawn, shoveling the snow, painting Bruce's new safe room and countless other tasks.

My dear sister Kathie has been a rock throughout the entire ordeal. She was always bringing food, encouragement, prayers and strength; heading up fund-raisers, cleaning the house (often with help from other sisters Dottie and Jill and sister-in law Gayle).

Kathie is also a full time neonatal intensive care nurse so she deals with pain and suffering every day. She has been incredible and to her I owe my sanity. She stayed overnight with Bruce in the hospital in Rochester when I was too exhausted to sleep. She kept telling me, "Bruce is going to make it," when the end seemed inevitable.

My parents and other siblings were also very supportive and donated a good portion of their own money to our fund-raisers. We owe them more than we can ever repay. We are also lucky to have some very dear friends who were there when we needed them most. Bruce was initially diagnosed when Syracuse was being blanketed with a terrible snowstorm.

I knew our friends, Jack and Liz were out on the town celebrating his birthday, but another friend Sue asked if she should contact them. I told her to leave a message for tomorrow. Within an hour, they were in the Emergency Room still dressed in their evening clothes and have been by our sides ever since. Liz has cooked for us, listened to me cry and been there for me so many times. Jack even spent the night with Bruce when Melissa, Kathie and I were not available.

He spent many hours walking the halls and sitting at Bruce's bedside in Rochester when Bruce was at his worst and it is a two and 1/2 hour trip over and back! Bruce is a lucky man to have so many loving family members and friends. Our church family and old college and high school friends also showed up when we needed them the most.

Bruce was placed on prayer chains from Texas to Alaska and most places in between. On some of the darkest days, we would receive cards from prayer chain members or family members that would bring sunlight into our room. I felt God's presence many times during this ordeal and He has been a constant comfort for me.

I first became interested in Environmental Medicine when our oldest daughter became ill almost twenty years ago.

I can't believe that in all that time and with all the documented successes this field of medicine has provided that more doctors are not practicing EM. It heals without surgery and without the use of toxic drugs. As a Registered Nurse, I witnessed the number of times that a drug would cause severe reactions only to be followed by more drugs to counteract the reactions of the first.

I suffered endless nightmares watching seemingly healthy people get worse every time I saw them. It is not easy for a person afflicted with an autoimmune related illness to accept the regimen that is required to get well and I had to essentially threaten Bruce before he would listen.

It is hard to give up your favorite foods and eating out and doing the things you enjoy on a daily basis to be replaced with rice and beans and lettuce and essentially tasteless foods. When we were in Texas, Bruce was so weak from the daily regimen that I had to do all the shopping and meal preparation while he slept.

I had to help him in and out of the car like he was a ninety-year-old man. It seemed like he was dying before my eyes. I spent countless hours developing a diet that met the requirements of the Environmental Health Center yet was palatable for Bruce.

The mission was clear - We had to get his toxic load down to prevent him from dying of toxic overload. The doctor and his staff were helpful, but it was clear that I would have to be the primary caregiver. If you are the spouse of an infected person, I urge you to take this responsibility seriously. I would be exhausted at the end of a day, but now that I have my husband back, I am eternally grateful.

The financial burden was overwhelming at times but I just decided that we were going to do whatever it took and we would figure out how to pay for it later. We had to sell our "dream home" after living in it for less than a year, but I did not hesitate when it meant saving his life.

Thankfully we had a fund-raiser hosted by our good friends, Mark and Karen that raised most of the money we needed to pay for the trip to Dallas. Mark even took time off from his busy schedule as the owner of a golf course to drive Bruce back to Texas after Melissa's wedding.

To the caretakers who read this, I offer this advice. I do not claim to be an expert in the field of Environment Medicine, but I want to add my personal recommendations to what Bruce has already said.

Read everything you can find about Environmental Medicine beginning with the excellent series by Dr. Sherry Rogers. If you read her books, you will know much more about how our environment is killing us than most doctors.

It is probably the most important thing you can do for your loved one and he or she will not have the strength to do it early on. They need every ounce of energy they have left just to stay alive. They will likely need regular blood transfusions and there is no getting around that one in the beginning.

Take control of your own destiny and do not rely solely on your doctor. As Dr. Rogers says, "You can heal yourself, but you have to figure it out on your own. No doctor, including me, is going to do it for you." Find a way to get your loved one tested for allergies and toxic exposure. Change his/her diet and return to natural, organically raised fruits and vegetables. Try the "grains, greens and beans" diet Dr. Rogers describes in her book, "The Cure Is in the Kitchen."

I know in my heart of hearts it is what is keeping him alive. This is what Bruce has done and continues to do. He is constantly reading and learning about his illness and alternative ways of dealing with it. He has always been driven with endless energy and the power of positive thinking.

Whether he calls himself a Jack-of-All-Trades, Bubba, Buster, Mister, the Rabbit Man or whatever, there is very little in life that he cannot do if he sets his mind to it. I am so proud of him and I continue to hope and pray that we will have another 33 plus years together.

Sue

* * * * *

A Message from Doctor Henry G. Bieler

"As a practicing physician for over fifty years, I have reached three basic conclusions as to the cause and cure of disease. This book is about those conclusions. The first is that the primary cause of disease is not germs.

Rather, I believe that disease is caused by a toxemia that results in cellular impairment and breakdown, thus paving the way for the multiplication and onslaught of germs.

My second conclusion is that in almost all cases the use of drugs in treating patients is harmful. Drugs often cause serious side effects, and sometimes even create new diseases. The dubious benefits they afford the patient are at best temporary. Yet the number of drugs on the market increases geometrically every year as each chemical firm develops its own variation of the compounds. The physician is indeed rare who can be completely aware of the potential danger from the side effects of all of these drugs.

My third conclusion is that disease can be cured through the proper use of correct foods. This Statement may sound deceptively simple, but I have arrived at it only after intensive study of a highly complex subject: colloid and endocrine chemistry. My conclusions are based on experimental and observational results, gathered through years of successfully treating patients.

Occasionally I have resorted to the use of drugs in emergency situations, but those times have been rare. Instead, I have sought to prescribe for my patients' illnesses antidotes that Nature has placed at their disposal. Far too many of these new "miracle" drugs are introduced with fanfare and then revealed as lethal in character, to be silently discarded for newer and more powerful drugs, which allegedly cure all the ills to which the flesh is heir.

I discarded drugs partly because I began to re-examine an old, old medical truism--that nature does the real healing, utilizing the natural defenses of the body. Under the proper conditions nature, if given the opportunity, is always the greatest healer. It is the physician's role to assist in this healing - to co-operate with nature's forces- to play a supporting role instead of star of the show. Nature does not follow Madison Avenue's "Feel Better Faster" but takes her time, slowly, as a tree grows, a little more each day. Nature never rushes to get a sick man or beast on his feet; she also demands a slow and steady convalescence. Sick animals rest or sleep and refuse all food until nature has healed them.

Isn't it proper, then, to expect that nature can do the same thing for the sick human if only she is given the opportunity? Because I believe this so deeply, I have been in disagreement with doctors who stuff the sick, exhausted man with powerful toxic drugs and then are forced to use other drugs to "remedy the remedy," as it were. Instead I "fast" the patient on simple vegetable broths or diluted fruit juices in order to give the exhausted body organs an opportunity to discharge their waste products and heal themselves."

Both excerpts are from "Food is Your Best Medicine" by Henry G. Bieler, M.D. -

A Message from Dr. Sherry Rogers

Paraphrased from the introduction to Wellness against All Odds by Sherry A. Rogers, M.D.

Dr. Rogers presents a strong case for an alternative approach to modern medicine based on her years of research into biochemistry reading of medical journals, courses attended and practical experience with thousands of patients. She asserts, "Cancer is not a chemotherapy deficiency", just as headaches are not caused by a lack of Darvon and Arthritis is not caused by a shortage of Motrin.

In nearly all cases, modern medicine is treating and masking the very symptoms that are trying to advise us that something is desperately wrong with what we are doing to our bodies. Toxins or stress or allergies or some physical ailment causes headaches. The modern treatment is to mask the symptom with drugs.

She has spent a lifetime researching the previously silent underground of patients from all over the world who are using alternative strategies to cure themselves of "un-diagnosable" or ""untreatable" conditions.

As she says, "It turns out that there are a number of natural and inexpensive program with which people have done the impossible."

Her most telling comment however is this: "the patient is the one who plays the major role in determining whether or not the patient gets well."

* * * * *

Chapter 8

A Trip to Rochester

The BMT Team Presents

Our next stop was Strong Memorial Hospital in Rochester for further testing and my journal included the following entry:

January 17, 2001

I was released from Community General on my own recognizance and had been cautioned to take it easy (as if I had the energy to try anything) and was now meeting with Jeff the Elder and his Nurse Practitioner, Kathy Klinger. There was evidently some doubt about the initial diagnosis and I would definitely be going to Rochester next week for additional testing.

Evidently The Elder's experience is in leukemia and the folks in Rochester have more experience in the disorders that appear less frequently. I also had my Human Leukocyte Antigens (HLA) typing done for comparison with siblings and signed forms allowing the results to be forwarded to the Bone Marrow Database.

I must admit the urgency of the actions being taken was definitely getting my attention. Hmmm

The Elder also prescribed Prednisone (Steroid) to help build my strength and left me with the hope that one of my siblings will match my HLA type; whatever that is.

* * * * *

Two weeks after my initial race to the ER, we were introduced to the Rochester Bone Marrow Transplant, "BMT Team" at Strong Memorial. My lead doctor was Jeff the Younger - Dr. Jeff Lancet who looked young enough to be my grandson. He was baby faced but very serious.

I later learned this serious nature is very common amongst Oncologists and Hematologists since they deal with death and life threatening illnesses on a very regular basis. Because they rarely can affect a lasting cure, they are very guarded in their dispensing of any good news and they maintain a very reserved manner so the patients realize the serious nature of their illnesses.

Upon learning of my situation, both sister Martha in Des Moines, Iowa and brother Greg in Minneapolis went immediately to their doctors and had the necessary HLA (Human Leukocyte Antigens) testing done. It took a few days to get the results, and in the end, they were not good HLA matches. My HLA characteristics were A2, A24, B7, B62 and Greg's were A1, A24, B8, B62, CW, and CW7. I never actually saw Martha's but was assured they were also not close enough.

According to Nurse Coordinator Sharon and Jeff the Younger this is not a good enough match and I would therefore be better off with a MUD (Matched Unrelated Donor). We will set that issue aside for now as we move on to considering other less dangerous options. Transplant donors and recipients are matched by certain tissue characteristics called HLA markers.

* * * * *

These molecules, which vary from person to person, are involved in the body's ability to distinguish its own cells from that of foreign invaders. When HLA markers closely match, unrelated tissues are more likely to be compatible. If they do not match, however, the recipient's immune system may reject the transplanted tissue.

Unfortunately, finding a good HLA match can be difficult, especially for people with rare tissue types or without any closely matched relatives. The most popular way to test for tissue compatibility is to take a blood sample and test it against a set of antibodies that react to HLA proteins, or antigens. If the match is not perfect, there is a danger of contracting Graft Versus Host Disease or GVHD.

According to the Johns Hopkins Oncology Center, Graft Versus Host Disease is really two different diseases. An early form of Graft-versus-Host disease is called acute Graft-versus-Host disease. It occurs immediately after the transplant when the white cells rise. A late form of Graft-versus-Host disease called chronic Graft-versus-Host disease can be even more serious often resulting in death or debilitating injuries. The signs and symptoms of these two diseases differ and will be discussed separately.

Acute Graft-versus-Host disease is caused by the T-lymphocyte, a type of white cell, when it recognizes the patient's body as being foreign. The T-lymphocytes are harvested with the bone marrow graft from the donor and transferred in the graft. T-lymphocytes normally help protect the body from bacteria, viruses, and fungus.

When a T-lymphocyte from the donor realizes it is in a new location, it attacks the host body seeing it as foreign and therefore a threat. The T-lymphocyte is able to recognize differences based on a set of genetic markers called Human Leukocyte Antigens (HLA). Although most patients and donors are matched as closely as possible for HLA markers, we know that there are many minor markers that differ between donors and patients, except when the patient and donor are identical twins.

Before a transplant, extensive typing of the donor and recipient take place to try to make sure that the donor and recipient are very close immunologically (i.e. have the same HLA type). Despite this typing we know that there are differences that we do not detect and that the T-lymphocyte in the donor graft are not capable of recognizing.

The disease that results from the T-cells attacking the patient is called Graft-versus-Host disease. Acute Graft-versus-Host disease usually occurs within the first three months following a transplant. T-cells present in the donor's bone marrow at the time of transplant attack the patient's skin, liver, stomach, and/or intestines.

The earliest sign of acute Graft-Versus-Host Disease is usually a skin rash that appears on the hand, feet, and face. The rash may spread to other parts of the body and develop into a general red rash similar to sunburn. Patients developing blistering skin disease have severe Graft-versus-Host disease.

Likewise, patients developing large amounts of watery or bloody diarrhea with cramping have severe Graft-versus-Host disease of the stomach and/or intestines. Jaundice, yellowing of the skin and eyes, is the usual indication that Graft-versus-Host disease involves the liver.

Graft-versus-Host disease is rated according to the severity of the rash, diarrhea, and/or jaundice. The more organs involved and the worse the symptoms, the worse the Graft-versus-Host disease.

Strong Memorial Hospital is one of about 12 Regional Cancer Centers with a Bone Marrow Transplant Unit and a staff of well-trained doctors and nurses with wide ranging experience treating blood related disorders such as Leukemia, MDS, cancers, and Aplastic Anemia - now my official diagnosis.

With Aplastic Anemia, a patient's bone marrow is hypo plastic which means it has a fewer number of blood forming cells than a normal person. The bone marrow essentially stops producing healthy blood cells.

The hallmark of Aplastic Anemia is the empty bone marrow and the reduced production of normal blood cells. Megakaryocytes (the immature cells that normally produce platelets) are either absent (replaced by fat) or are malformed. Cells bearing the CD34 antigen (discussed in the chapter on Cellular Research) are virtually absent in the blood and marrow of patients with Aplastic Anemia.

The so called pluripotent cells (precursors to megakaryocytes) are also present in much lower volume than is normal and even the stem cells (the cells that begin the whole process) are present in a reduced number.

In the book of Genesis, it would sound like this: The stem cells beget the pluripotent (or multipotent) cells; the pluripotent cells beget the procrythroblasts, myleoblasts, lymphoblasts, monoblasts, and megakaryoblasts.

The procrythroblasts beget the megakaryocytes and the megakaryocytes beget the etc. ad nauseum.

And they all come from the house and lineage of the stem cell.

For a much more clear understanding, see the haematopoeisis chart in the Cellular Research chapter.

With Myelodysplasia, there are a normal number of cells being produced, but they are malformed so the T cells are destroying them before they enter the blood stream.

Regional Centers That Have Performed Bone Marrow Transplants

Center	Location	Year Started	Total Number of BMT's	Number Per Year
Hutchins	Seattle, WA	1973	7582	281
Stanford	Stanford, CA	1986	2185	156
Sloan	New York	1973	3599	133
Dan Farber	Boston, MA	1972	2679	96
Strong	**Rochester, NY**	**1989**	**1040**	**95**
Johns Hopkins	Baltimore, MD	1968	2942	92
Loyola	Chicago, IL	1986	1262	90
Roswell Park	Buffalo, NY	1991	647	72
Mayo	Rochester, MN	1982	991	55
Kaiser	Los Angeles, CA	1981	900	47
SUNY Upstate	Syracuse, NY	1992	372	47
Rush Memorial	Chicago, IL	1984	704	44

With the HLA discussion now behind us, we moved on to considering the other treatment options but not before I was subjected to two more Bone Marrow Biopsies by new "friend" Lucy. She was actually very good at this procedure that consists of literally drilling into my hip to extract a small chunk of bone.

Following the results of the biopsies, I was advised that I would likely be admitted for one of the less invasive treatments.

Within a few days, Lucy informed me that the preliminary diagnosis of Severe Aplastic Anemia had now been confirmed. SAA means my bone marrow has stopped producing blood cells properly and they are not being allowed to enter my blood stream.

My T cells are destroying the stem cells before they can mature and be released into the blood. My bone marrow is hypo plastic, which means it contains a low number of blood forming stem cells. In MDS, the cells are being produced but they are malformed. The treatment protocol for both is very similar, so the disease is not as important as the treatment strategy.

They will schedule me for admission to Strong Memorial within the next two weeks for Immunosuppressant Therapy. This treatment is designed to suppress the T Cells from destroying my healthy cells, which are being allowed to enter the blood stream. Alternative treatments are Antithymocyte Globulin Therapy ATG (Horse Serum) and Anti-Human Interleukin ALG (Rabbit Serum)

* * * * *

The intensity of the past several days and the weeks to come were overwhelming. Time stood still and then suddenly it raced huge bursts. My life became one long series of contradictions.

People entered and left my life so quickly that names and faces blurred. Others made an impression that will last me the rest of life.

The curious phenomenon of reduced blood flow at times dulled my senses and at other times heightened my state of alert. My heart often felt like it would pound itself out of my chest as it tried to keep up with the demands of my mind and body.

Aplastic Anemia patients rarely feel much pain or even feel sick for that manner. Acquaintances often comment on how great we look and we sometimes have the uncomfortable feeling that they think we are faking this whole thing to get a little attention.

All the while, we are slowly dying from a bizarre illness in which our immune system attacks our own bodies - not unlike the dreaded Acquired Immune Deficiency Syndrome (AIDS) associated with HIV.

With Aplastic Anemia, our body incorrectly determines that our malformed blood cells are potentially dangerous to our bodies and destroys these cells before they can enter our blood stream and accomplish their assignments. Red Blood Cells carry oxygen to our organs, White Blood Cells fight infection and Platelets provide the clotting function so vital in stopping the inevitable bleeding associated with even minor scrapes and bruises.

We learn that we could literally bleed to death from even the smallest cut or bruise. We are advised to avoid all contact sports, stay away from crowds and seriously curtail our lifestyles.

Except for the hidden bruises and our yellow pallor, we appear very normal on the outside while on the inside our immune system is destroying our malformed cells. We rarely suffer any real pain but this lack of pain can unfortunately allow us to press on until the diagnosis is only determined post mortem.

* * * * *

Included on the Bone Marrow Transplant Team are two of my new best friends, Lucy and Sharon. Lucy is a Nurse Practitioner and Sharon is a RN and the BMT coordinator.

Sharon will ultimately arrange for my hospitalizations and become my advocate within the hospital. My family and I also meet with social worker Mike and discuss the issues of family finances, depression and how to emotionally deal with this dreaded intrusion entry in our lives.

Mike also becomes a trusted advocate and my part time "shrink" as I begin to face the realities of what Aplastic Anemia has done to my life. He takes us on a tour of the state of the art Transplant Center that includes a completely isolated floor with its own ventilation system to prevent germs entering the environment from the outside.

They also warned us that all the potential treatments and especially a bone marrow transplant are very high-risk procedures. They are all very helpful and for the first time I began to wonder what all this is going to cost. Will insurance cover everything? How will we come up with the money for all these treatments? Thank God Sue has good insurance but I still wonder if it will be enough.

Yes, Mike and Mary assure us the insurance covers the medical bills, but what about the rest of our lives? We had become very accustomed to not paying much attention to what things cost. We went out to dinner 3-4 times per week and enjoyed a very comfortable lifestyle. My find is again racing with the thought of how this dreaded illness is disrupting our lives.

This was all about to change big time, as my earning power immediately dropped to zero! Because I was self-employed, there was no two-week notice, no severance pay, and no cushion whatsoever. Melissa came through like a commando and kept the business afloat, but we were about to face some very real changes in our lives.

Following the initial trip to Rochester, I began compiling my own knowledge base and started with this entry to my journal:

Antilymphocyte Globulin (ALG) is a Rabbit Serum designed to suppress my immune system. I guess I'll be the Rabbit Man! According to an article distributed by Aplastic Anemia & MDS International Foundation, "The generally accepted thinking about aplastic anemia is that the patient's immune system is reacting against the bone marrow, interfering with its ability to make blood cells. Immunosuppressive drugs are believed to counter this problem by reducing the immune response, allowing the bone marrow to once again make blood cells."

* * * * *

We will be seeing this entire group at least monthly for the next year and I appreciated the cohesive care resulting from their efforts, including the friendly group in Jeff the Elder's office and my "girl friends" at the "Home Tonight" unit at Community General Hospital. I have become a regular in all three places and they all treat me with great kindness and understanding. I have come to cherish the real caregivers in our medical system and they have my heartfelt thanks.

* * * * *

The BMT Team ultimately answered all our questions in the original and subsequent visits to Rochester. The biggest relief came when Mary and Sharon confirmed that nearly all of our direct medical expenses would most likely be covered by insurance or various grants that are available to them as a teaching and research hospital.

Chapter 9

"Oh, My God"

A Trip to Medical Hell

Thanks to a "local" anesthetic, I was acutely aware of everything around me when I heard the surgeon say,

"Oh, my God, I missed", followed by some light laughter and his assistant saying, "It won't kill him, it's only his heart."

Very funny guys! This was my life and my heart you are joking about and I didn't find this one bit funny! I could actually feel them sticking a wire prod into my heart for the insertion of a Central Line Hickman Catheter. The catheter became a primary element for delivering meds, extracting blood and the infusion of platelets and packed red blood cells during my first long hospitalization since my original diagnosis.

This initial catheter experience was by far the worst but over the next eighteen months, I would be subjected to several similar episodes. I now bear several scars in my chest to remind me that I will probably never be completely normal again.

Don't get me wrong, it certainly was nice avoiding the constant poking associated with Intravenous (IV) blood draws and medicine infusions, but I definitely could have done without the insertion of metal tubes into my heart, chest, and arms.

Imagine having three six inch plastic tubes hanging out of your chest. That is a Triple Lumen Hickman (named for the person who invented it) Catheter. It is in fact a very ugly thing that is directly attached to my aorta but it does save me from being poked for an IV every time I needed blood drawn. Having never been hospitalized before this was an eye opening experience. It's very different being the one in the bed vs. visiting someone else.

I later teased my younger friends that I was an alien and had to "plug in" every night to be recharged. (This was not that far from the truth as daily infusions of one kind or another became routine.)

The Hickman procedure was referred to as minor surgery and in fact was conducted under local anesthesia but I certainly didn't enjoy it very much. After some minor prepping, they shot some Lydocaine into my chest and then before I knew it they were poking around my heart and sticking this long plastic tube in me. See the picture below so you're not surprised like I was!

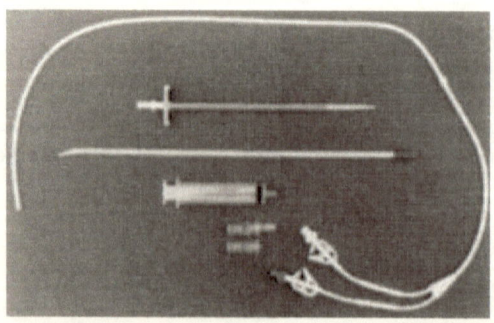

Catheters - What to Expect

During the term of my hospitalizations and transfusions, I experienced several different strategies for the infusion of blood products, withdrawal of blood samples and delivery of medications.

Most people are familiar with the peripheral IV line that you see hanging out of a patients arm during almost any hospitalization. Since this requires a new insertion every two or three days, a person's veins eventually collapsed or become unusable.

The catheter or PICC line was invented as an alternative to these multiple IV "pokes."

I am back to a "new type" of PICC line according to the nurse practitioner who put it in. She had a great time poking around trying to get it inserted. My arm looks and feels like a punching bag. I feel like a much-abused guinea pig. This is now my fourth catheter in a little over a year.

I have now been the proud recipient of three types of catheters so I can speak from practical experience and hopefully warn some of you about pluses/minuses and dos and don'ts regarding central lines.

As described above, my first experience was with the Hickman Long Term Triple Lumen Tunneled Catheter - Hickman was the inventor and "triple lumen" refers to the number of tubes that would ultimately be hanging out of my chest. It's kind of like plumbing - Hot, Cold and Warm with separate "faucets" for each.

In practice I was thankful for the multiple ports because there were times when I was receiving blood in one port, medications in the other and the third was reserved for blood draws.

This first device was installed via a surgical procedure in February of 2001 and lasted for about 8 months before becoming infected. This was by far the most painful and invasive as it required two incisions but it did last me a long time and helped avoid numerous butchered IV insertions. (My arms had become black and blue from all the needle pokes during my initial hospitalization and multiple transfusions.

They began by injecting a small amount of the local anesthetic and then made two relatively small cuts, one in my neck just above the collarbone and the other in my chest. They then "fished" a wire down through my vein and directly into the left atrium of my heart.

This is not as scary as it sounds, but I would have appreciated knowing what to expect before the procedure. Plastic tubing that becomes the permanent IV tube then follows the wire. Finally they "tunnel" down from the insertion point in your neck to a permanent mounting place on your chest, attach the claves (little blue connectors which provide a heparin lock to prevent leakage and little plastic clamps which are a further safeguard.)

The whole procedure took about an hour from start to finish and if I were to have this done again, I would opt for "real" anesthesia rather than the local. It was not a pleasant experience. I had some rather annoying pain for a couple of days afterwards and then it became like an old friend.

I "flushed the ports" on a daily basis with the 10 cc's of saline. This procedure keeps the lines "patent" or able to draw back and forth. I also had to change the tagaderm (clear vinyl patch) dressing on a regular basis. After several months, the stitching used to secure the catheter to my chest became very irritable and ultimately became so infected that I landed in the hospital with a sepsis (blood) infection that caused rigors (shaking), severe chills and a fever of over 105 degrees.

This was definitely no fun and landed me in the hospital for about a week. As a result, my Hickman was removed. This procedure had to be done by a surgeon but it was less painful then the insertion and was performed in my room rather than in a surgical area.

I then had a Peripherally Inserted Central Catheter (PICC) installed in the fleshy part of my left arm just below the elbow. This was by far the least painful but also the most useless device. If they suggest a PICC, run the other direction. Mine only lasted about two months, was constantly in the way and ultimately pulled completely out.

In fairness to the PICC, my "stat lock" got wet shortly after the insertion and none of the people who looked at the line knew enough to replace the stat lock (a very sticky butterfly type bandage that locks the line in place on your arm). I subsequently learned (while having my Hohn installed) that immediate replacement of the stat lock might have prevented the line from pulling out.

My final experience involved a "semi-permanent" device inventor). The installation procedure was performed by experience but less painful.

called a Hohn Catheter (again named for the a radiologist and was similar to the Hickman

It required only a single insertion point near the collarbone and does not normally require suturing. (The doctor made the decision at the end depending on how well the insertion went). In my case, they decided the stat lock would suffice.

It is more exposed than the other two devices and it looks like a Frankenstein tubes hanging out of my neck.

The Hohn catheter lasted about a week and when it came out we discovered that it had barely enough tubing to make it from the insertion point to my heart. I'm not sure if it was a botched installation or the device itself but I would certainly question anyone who recommended this device.

Closing comments - be very careful in the first few days to not get the "site" (insertion point) wet and then try to keep it covered with saran wrap or a "baggie" when you shower. Moisture under the bandage is bad news! If it gets wet, change it immediately. I'm pretty sure that I contributed to my sepsis experience by letting mine get wet (got careless after a while). Also be sure that you or anyone who changes the dressing thoroughly (20-30 second scrub) washes their hands and wears gloves. My wife (RN) tells me that the gunk under your fingernails is the number one cause of sepsis infections.

* * * * *

I remember muttering "Oh, my God" myself the night before when my new friend Dr. Camille Aboud declared,

"You will never be normal again."

Dr. Aboud was my admitting doctor for what I now refer to as my trip thru medical hell. This is by no means a reflection on the University of Rochester Medical Center or any of its staff, but the Snafu's associated with my initial admission quickly went from bad to worse.

Prior to the "Oh, My God" experience, I had some interesting encounters with hospital administration. First, I was admitted in the evening after all the regular staff had departed so my admissions person was a bit, shall we say, lethargic. Here I was, about to undergo some unknown life-threatening procedure and she was filing her nails and treating me like I was an interruption.

After discussing the alternatives and consulting with other staff members, Jeff the Younger had decided that I needed to be admitted for my first round of "ATG". I will tell you more about that later, but for now I was not real happy with the way my treatment experience was progressing.

After about 90 minutes, my nail filing friend finally figured out where I was supposed to go and I was wheeled into a room with a young man who barely acknowledged my presence and was continually flipping through the channels of his overbearing television.

At the time, I was not a very tolerant person but this was really too much. I had been given a tour of an entirely different area of the hospital - the Bone Marrow Treatment Center, where everyone had a private, environmentally controlled room. I had been told that I should not be exposed to germs, since my White Blood Cell count was so low.

So here I was in a double room in the middle of a unit filled with all kinds of sick people!

I think Jeff the Younger had some personal issues of his own happening at that time because he was gone for a couple of weeks while I was in the hospital. Meanwhile, I was exhausted and knew that I needed some rest, so I requested a transfer to another room. I think Sue had to leave to make arrangements for a place to stay, so here I was stuck with the "Channel Flicker."

Dr. Aboud is of Lebanese ancestry. He is a very interesting fellow in his mid-50's I would guess, but certainly no picture of health himself. He is overweight, stressed out and a workaholic. He appears to rely heavily on the chocolate and other junk food available at the nurse's station in the wee hours of the morning.

During my visit I saw him at all kinds of weird hours and know that he must have pulled several 24 hours shifts without any real rest. Take my admission for example: I showed up about 5:00 PM, was admitted about 7:00 and don't remember seeing "Camille" until probably 8:00 that night. He popped in just long enough to utter his comforting news about my future state of normalcy and then disappeared for several hours.

I didn't know it yet, but he spent the next several hours in a non-stop effort developing a plan of attack. As it turns out, the Younger had to leave town rather unexpectedly without giving Camille much to work with. As luck would have it, my primary care person, Nurse Practitioner Lucy Wedow was also not on duty that week so Camille really didn't have much to work with.

I assume he must have had to track down my chart from their offices in another wing of the hospital and develop his own plan of attack based on the transcription notes of the Younger.

He first had to determine what exactly was wrong with me, what he intended to do about it and then had to track down the drugs he would use to treat me. I guess rabbit serum is not something you find lying around on every street corner? I didn't get a real warm and fuzzy feeling when he asked me about my diagnosis. It was pretty clear that he had not been properly briefed and it was also very clear that I had not been admitted to one of the special rooms that had been showcased in my earlier tour of the Bone Marrow Transplant Unit by Social Worker, Mike Ellis. Looking back, we should have checked out immediately and gone back to Syracuse, but I was too sick and Sue was too distraught to be thinking very clearly.

"Bluce, he said in his heavy Lebanese accent, "ju vill, at some point, get very, very sick. Ju must believe me on dis, because I have seen it many times before. Just ven ju tink ju are OK, ju vill get hit very hard."

He went on to tell me that the treatment protocol they would use was first developed in Italy and he had been in consultation with other doctors who had used this particular regimen. It is a protocol fully supported by the National Institute of Health (NIH) and in fact according to Dr. Neil Young, it is the first effort that should be attempted for someone who does not have a matched sibling donor for a Bone Marrow Transplant.

* * * * *

Sue later reported that she was able to arrange for a room, at the Ronald McDonald House, during my first night of the "Oh my God" visit. It turned out to be a very nice safe haven for her and Melissa on a couple of occasions so we have a new respect for the Golden Arches!

After numerous discussions with several staff people, I was finally moved into another room with another obviously very sick person. That is when Sue pretty much lost it. She demanded to speak to the nurse manager and we were finally moved into a private room in another section. It really helped that Sue knew her way around a hospital and how to work her way up the chain of command.

The next day I was officially declared "neutropenic" (White Blood Cell count less than 1000) which meant I should not be exposed to any germs whatsoever, yet the night before I was shuttled back and forth and up and down the hallway exposed to all kinds of germs.

Now, everyone who entered my room was requested to wear a mask and gloves. I was in "reverse isolation." I was not a threat to others, but they were a threat to me. Jack began referring to me as the "Bubble Boy."

Besides being neutropenic, I was very weak and virtually everything I tried to do was an effort. To comprehend the extent of my debilitating weakness, listen to the simple exercise of getting to the bathroom while in the hospital for the first time. In the old me, it was a virtually unconscious act. The "new me" actually had to plan the effort. Where was the bathroom? What would I encounter on the way? How did I avoid tripping over my IV or chair on the way?

OK - ready to stand up. I no longer bounced out of my chair. Instead I balanced myself and did it in stages like I was eighty years old. I had to lift myself up, stop to regain my balance and push myself out of the chair or bed. Next, I had to position my IV tubing so as not to run over them on the way.

Then I had to reach down (an effort in itself) and unplug the IV power cord. It took far more energy than I could believe just to pull the cord from the wall outlet. I then shuffled down the hall, entered and did my business (took about three times longer than my previous unconscious effort). I was by now completely out of breath, so I needed to rest before beginning my twenty-step journey back to the safety of my bed.

Arriving back at my bed, I faced the difficult challenge of having to plug the cord back into the wall. It was actually a difficult thing to do (plugging a cord into the wall!). I accomplished this huge feat and finally settled in contemplate my next adventure. My hands were trembling, my heart was racing and I was now even weaker than an hour ago because I used up a goodly amount of the red blood cells that had been generously donated to me by a stranger – just getting to the bathroom!

My body will use them up, but not replenish them and so I was fighting a seemingly endless and un-winnable battle - the more I tried to do even the simplest exercise, the faster I burned blood cells and increased my fatigue and weakness.

This is not a "woe is me" story, it is simply the realization that for the first time in my life, there was little or nothing I could do to affect the outcome of my situation.

I was literally powerless and for someone who had prided himself on being able to do just about anything (from building a house and understanding everything about it to teaching myself how to be a power user of computers and launching three businesses, this was extremely difficult to accept).

I remember a very nice admitting nurse who gave me a chart explaining how the blood cells are produced and the difference between stem cells, T cells, etc. She also started me on "pre-meds" of Solumedrol, Celebrex, Protonic, Folic Acid, Dipluran and Cyclosporine.

I was also started on growth agents of EPO to stimulate growth of red blood cells and G-CSF for White Blood Cells and Platelets. I took more pills in one day than I had previously taken in my whole life!

Dr. Aboud explained my diagnosis more thoroughly and again reiterated that I would probably never be 100% of my old self. The best we could hope for with this strategy was to put the disease into remission and maybe I would return to 75% of my old self. I must realize that I have a chronic disease that is not going to go away! My T cells (Lymphoblasts) are attacking my White Blood Cells, Red Blood Cells and Platelets because they are malformed.

The therapy was designed to suppress this activity and if successful would reduce my dependence on transfusions. At the time of my admission to Strong Memorial, I was receiving platelets every five to seven days and blood every ten to fourteen days. Once admitted, I received platelets almost every day – sometimes twice a day and red blood cells every two-three days.

I was again advised there was a strong chance that I would have serum sickness of fevers, tremors, rashes, etc. so they gave me many prophylactic drugs designed to reduce the serum sickness.

I was also administered a desensitization procedure to determine if I had any allergies. An immunization team scratched my skin seven or eight places and inserted a minute amount of penicillin and other meds to see if my skin would react. There were no reactions so my life long belief that I was allergic to penicillin proved to me incorrect.

By February 9th, with my new catheter firmly in place and the allergy testing completed, it was determined that I was good to go for the ALG treatment. Bring on the rabbit!

It was administered over a four-day period and each dose took about five hours. It was delivered pretty much like any other IV drug. Hang it on the pole, connect it to a port and let it flow.

I had a bit of a flushed face near the end, but day one was otherwise uneventful.

First dose of rabbit serum about 6:00 PM with nurse Jen

On day two, I was declared fully neutropenic (white blood cell count below 1.0) and placed on a restricted diet

– No fresh fruit or vegetables or salad to minimize exposure to bacteria. Everyone who entered my room had to wash their hands, wear gloves and a mask. I was in reverse isolation. If I left my room, I had to wear a mask and be careful not to touch walls, railings etc.

They were drawing my blood twice a day –once about 4:00 in the morning and then again about 4:00 in the afternoon. I received two units of blood and five unites of platelets on both days two and three.

On day three my blood pressure rose to 160/100 from its norm of 120/80 and my pulse dropped to 43 beats per minute from its norm of 65. I experienced chest pain and shortness of breath so they stopped the ATG about half way through. They gave me another set of premeds (Benadryl, Tylenol and a hydrocortisone shot) and finished the dose.

I had difficulty sleeping that night so they gave me some Halycion about 1:30. This is the first time in my life I had taken anything to help me sleep. I felt "drugged" the next morning.

On day 4 (February 12) I received the last of my ATG treatments and I guess it accomplished it stated goal, because my white blood cell count fell to .1. Platelets were at 14 so received platelets for the fourth day in a row.

The next ten days were uneventful except for one morning I woke up with numbness in my left arm and shoulder. I was unable to lift my arm above my shoulder. I tried exercising it but it stayed that way for several days.

Little did I know it at the time, but that was minor compared to what happened next. Starting on about day 15 or sixteen (February 25) I got hit by a truck. Dr. Aboud had promised me I would get sick and he was not wrong.

It started with heart palpitations and before it was over, I had chest pains, shortness of breath, edema (swelling of joints), and insomnia. I began to lose strength and it got so bad I could not even get out of bed to use the bathroom. I had my first experience with learning how to use the bedpan and urinal. What fun!

I lost the use of my legs and my whole right side was semi-paralyzed for several days. I was pretty well out of it for several days. When I finally recovered my senses, I had completely lost the use of my right arm. I could not even lift it off the bed and was pretty frightened that it would stay that way.

Dr. Aboud arranged for a physical therapist to help me with some special exercises. I started very slowly but by the time I was released, I could at least raise my arm again.

The ALG treatment had successfully wiped out my immune system and I was hospitalized for 4 weeks while my body reacted to the serum ("serum sickness") and then began rebuilding itself.

Thank God I had my wife, daughters and friends around. The caregivers at Strong were fantastic and my core group has been great. They helped make it bearable and I realized how important it was to have family, friends and caretakers.

The serum sickness consisted of fevers, joint pain, insomnia and some other generally ugly side effects. The most debilitating side effect was the loss of feeling in my right arm and shoulder.

I was on a full regimen of "prophylactic medication" designed to prevent more serious effects. I tracked my blood cell counts from the beginning and continue to do so today.

Tracking platelets became my life's mission. I didn't even know what a platelet was five months ago and now I think about them every day. In preparation for my discharge, I was weaned off all my meds with the exception of the Cyclosporine (suppress the immune system) twice a day and the Diflucan, an anti-fungal.

I also received a growth factor shot (neuritis) once a day and of course have to "flush my ports" every day with saline.

It was during this first visit that, for the first time in my life, I felt as though I had lost control of everything. I was completely dependent on others and this was not normal for me. Since I could no longer control the more important aspects of my life, I became obsessed with trying to control the few things that I could.

I drove everyone crazy with my requests for bringing things from home trying to simulate home. I wanted a CD player. I needed my guitar. I needed my computer. Bring me more books to read. Please buy me the AEBIZ business plan so I can work on it in my spare time.

Unplug the phone so I can rest. Get me an extension cord and a phone extension so I can have everything where I need it.

Fluff up my pillows. No, not that way - like this. Oh, my God, what a pain I must have been. Thankfully everyone endured my lunacy and by the time I was finally released, we had to rent a U haul trailer to get everything out of my room.

By March 9, I was ready to go home. It had been a month since my admission and although I was still very weak, I badgered the doctors until they finally arranged for my discharge late in the afternoon. There was another blizzard brewing and I did not want to be stuck in Rochester for another three or four days.

Melanie was stuck in the back seat with all my accumulated junk and could barely move for the almost two hour trip in terrible weather. Sue endured my telling her how to drive (what a pain I was once again) and I fretted and worried like a frightened old man.

On returning home, I was set up with home care to check my catheter and draw blood every two days. I was too weak to travel so this was a welcome relief. I settled into a routine of platelets every week and blood every two weeks waiting to see if the ALG would work. I could not drive myself, so Melissa became my trusted taxi driver for the transfusions. I was told that the ALG could take up to six months before it showed the desired results (normal blood counts).

On March 15, Sue, Melissa and I made the trip to Rochester for a follow up visit with Jeff the Younger and the BMT team. They reiterated how important it was for the ALG protocol to work because a transplant for someone my age and size was extremely high risk.

I was assured that the number of transplants I received should not be an issue (I had read that too many transfusions can be problematic as my body will build up antibodies to the foreign entities); I was still concerned about that.

We agreed that my thresholds for transfusion would be 10 for platelets and 25 for hematocrits. I returned to Syracuse to wait it out, continue with home care treatment and wonder what to do next.

The "Oh My God" experience was finally behind me.

Chapter 10

A New Routine Begins

BMT, ALG, CGH & HOACNY

April 2, 2001

By early April of 2001 I felt well enough to discontinue my home care treatment. Before discharging me, the BMT team had arranged for daily visits by a home health care nurse who checked my vitals and helped me with IV meds (Vancomycin antibiotic and others as necessary)

I actually felt well enough to start back to a semi-normal work schedule. I traveled to Albany and Batavia and worked in Syracuse 2-3 days per week. I was usually pretty strong in the AM but by 3:00 would start to wear down.

The mid-April checkup with Dr. Lancet was mostly uneventful. There were no indications that anything had worked yet, but I agreed to be patient.

Additional visits yielded the same results and my counts continued to hover at very low levels. When I was not traveling to Rochester, I was visiting Dr. Kirshner's HOACNY office and going to the Home Tonight Center at Community General Hospital for weekly platelet transfusions and bi-weekly blood transfusions.

* * * * *

The following entries are a summary of my journal from May and June of 2001:

I continue to be weak which is very frustrating - things I used to take for granted like turning a screwdriver were virtually impossible between weakness and shakes from the Prednisone. It's comical to watch me try to work a mouse.

I want to get off the steroids and will be weaned over the next week or so. I guess it's not good to stop cold turkey, as there can be some damaging results.

The effort to be declared officially disabled by the Social Security Administration is moving along. They told me last time I called that I had been "fast tracked" and should expect to hear by September. Supposedly the payments will be retroactive to July for about $1600/month.

This would definitely take some of the financial pressure off. Also had a good talk with Art from ARAmatic regarding the possibility of helping out part time if able and renewed talks with an old friend from Digital regarding possible opportunity with a company he has started. Although it may be a nice long-term opportunity, it does not appear that it will generate any income in the short term and that is what we need right now.

My old golf buddy and owner of the Links at Sunset Ridge, Mark Clark has offered to host a benefit golf tournament in August. He says we should generate at least $10,000.

Son-in-law Mike has been a blessing. He helps out with all the physical stuff I am no longer able to do. I never thought I could become so helpless so quickly. I remember my Dad being so frustrated when this happened to him so many years ago. In addition to losing physical strength, he also could no longer think clearly. I am experiencing the same inability to complete a thought and it is very frustrating.

Mike finally seems to have the pool working after several false attempts with help from friends Mark, Ray and Jack. It is a real pain! I get frustrated when I am unable to do what used to be simple things like turning a couple of pipe wrenches against each other. I have limited upper body and arm strength. I try to exercise and am completely exhausted from even the slightest exertion.

My body is really a joke! I am putting on weight and my face looks fat from the Prednisone and there doesn't appear to be anything I can do to deal with the lack of energy and strength. Even a short walk leaves me exhausted. I am also fighting severe leg cramps. They are really bizarre. I have experienced cramps before, but usually in the muscles of the calf or thigh. These are in my toes and on the tops of my shins – very strange! Melissa bought me an early father's day present of a foot bath/massage that really helped.

It's like the song says, "Some Days are Diamonds, and Some Days are Stones". Just when it appeared that things might stabilize, all my counts tanked again. The mood swings and bouncing back and forth between hope and despair is very frustrating for me. I have always been very optimistic and able to do things for myself. It is hard to be so dependent on others and not able to shake this thing.

However, whenever I get feeling sorry for myself, I look around at people that are a lot worse than I and I dig in again. I am not going to sit around and let this thing get me! I will become my own one-man research team and figure out what the heck can be done about this thing

On the good news front, we have a date for the Golf Benefit It will be held on August 18th and Sue, Mark and Karen, Kathie and Laverne, John and Nancy Knowlton and Ron and Sue Richer will go to work getting sponsors, players and donations.

After a couple of really good days with friends and just keeping up with things, I got some kind of infection and crashed again. Golly, gee whiz this is fun! I guess this is probably a milder form of the serum sickness.

A visit to HOACNY revealed that indeed my counts had crashed again. Platelets are at a near all-time low of 6,000 and White Blood Cells are at a very dangerous level of 1000. Hematocrits are 24,000.

I will receive platelets immediately and will have to wait until tomorrow for blood, as the Red Cross is low on my required type. This makes me realize how dependent I am on others and just how tenuous my situation. Regarding the infection, I will be placed on yet another new medication called Ceftriaxone for e-coli.

After the blood products and a few days on the new medication, I began to feel better but this up and down stuff is no fun!

Sue and I have done a lot of reading lately on chemical sensitivities, diet, etc. and are going to again try a low carbohydrate, macrobiotic diet. I have also decided to more clearly document what I am doing in hopes that it may be of help to others.

I will attempt to be as factual and objective as possible and include research into immunology, the blood system, immunotherapy, multiple chemical sensitivities, environmental allergies, etc.

As more time goes by and I continue to see no real improvement, I begin to be concerned about my options. No matter what I am told, I continue to be concerned about the number of transfusions I am receiving. Every transfusion is an opportunity for infection and the introduction an infectious disease.

My age is also definitely working against me as I have been told that most centers will not perform BMT's on people over 55. If I am going to have a transplant, I should request it pretty soon. It has now been six months since my formal diagnosis and it is likely that I had the illness for at least a year before that as I could feel myself getting progressively weaker over a long period of time.

I still feel pretty lousy even after the transfusions but am especially weak just prior to the next transfusion. I used to get a surge of energy after transfusion but this has not been the case for the last two.

Now I wonder if they will become even less effective as time goes on. So far, I have received a total of forty-three transfusions. I now struggle to lift twenty pounds. I vividly recall throwing around bales of hay and eighty pound bags of fertilizer like it was nothing – hmmm funny I would remember the fertilizer thing since that may have been a culprit in my current dilemma. I used to handle the stuff all day long with no mask or any type of protection.

I drove a little Melroe Bobcat front-end loader up and down this huge open pole barn with dust from fertilizer everywhere. Granted, this was a long time ago but I had at least two years continued exposure working in the fertilizer plant. I breathed that stuff in all summer long. I wonder if others who worked in similar environments have Aplastic Anemia or similar illnesses. One of the members of Aplastic Central is convinced that exposure to Benzene was a cause of his illness and he is starting a lawsuit.

After the most recent transfusion episode on Monday and Tuesday, I tried to work a half day Wednesday and pretty much tanked about 2:00. Thrusday I was off to Rochester for a CBC and growth shots. That's a pretty typical week!

June 28, 2001 - The Roller Coaster Ride Continues

After feeling absolutely lousy and discouraged yesterday, today was unbelievably good! I met with my Rochester Nurse Practitioner Lucy and we discussed what to do if the current treatment strategy does not work. She informed me that they were already considering me for a clinical trial and would be working to get me into a T Cell Depletion protocol as part of an unrelated transplant.

The T Cell depletion strategy greatly reduces the risk of GVHD and improves the odds of survival to 75%. She pointed me to some information and promised to send more. We will be researching and updating each other over the next few days. (As a side note, it is extremely important that all you patients out there become active in your own treatment strategy.)

Melissa and I then worked with a customer and everything went like clockwork. I'm still at it and feeling almost normal. What gives with this thing called AA anyways?? I really don't understand the ups and downs.

We stopped in at the Medical Library at Strong and discovered some real secrets on how to research the illness. Lucy will be putting me back on Vanko (takes 1.45 hrs. in the AM and same in PM vs. Ceftriaxone which takes only about 10 minutes. Oh well, it gives me time to update the web site.

* * * * *

I had several very bad reactions (hives and swelling) before we arrived at a pre-med combination of Tylenol, Benadryl and the hydrocortisone shot delivered at least 20-30minutes prior to my transfusion. Although they were very good and conscientious, I had to be my own advocate in telling the nurses what to do and when.

With all the transfusions going on, Sue inquired about Liver Enzymes and something called bilirubin? It sounded like some guy to me so I had a hard time keeping up. Apparently my fatigue and constant jaundiced look were of concern and I would be tested for iron overload.

Turns out my "ferritin" (iron) level was a whopping 2500 vs. the norm of 250. Wow, someone should start mining the stuff from by body! Yes, Bubba you are officially jaundiced and Sue says it is because I have too much iron and my system is not properly breaking down and disposing of dead red blood cells.

The number of blood transfusions I have received has resulted in a buildup or iron from the blood of others and my system is unable to remove it on its own. I will begin receiving something called Desferol to combat this build up.

Desferol is an "iron chelator" which means it helps to remove or chelate excess iron from my body.

And speaking of fatigue, I attempted to mow a flat front lawn that used to seem like no big deal and was actually looking forward to it as a way to get some exercise. After only about ten minutes, I was flat out exhausted and had all I could do to get the mower to a safe place and me into a chair. It took me 30 minutes to restore my breathing back to normal!

I had serious bout with diarrhea was asked to provide a specimen (I just love to talk medical talk – not!) and given a prescription for Flagil for Diarrhea/CDEF. Once the results were returned, I had pretty much cleared up and it was confirmed that I had CDEF (A more serious version of the infection I had earlier.)

In late May, we pretty much agreed that ALG treatment number one was not successful so we began making arrangements for a second attempt.

A typical visit to the Hematology Center

While writing the book, I received an inquiry from a website visitor wondering about the blood testing, so decided to offer the following description:

In my visit to the HOACNY today, I asked if I could "follow my blood" through the lab just to see what happens. They were very accommodating and I was actually surprised at how simple the process was and the short amount of involved.

After logging me in on the computer, the first step is to get my sample. This is really quite painless. A Phlebotomist puts a syringe on my arm just above the elbow, slides a little butterfly needle (not much bigger than a small household needle) into a vein, starts some idle conversation and before I know it, she has two or three little test tubes (vials) filled with my precious liquid.

She sends me back to the waiting room (this time I stayed to see the process) and they place the vials on a little vibrating table to keep it from coagulating. When it is my turn, a technician inserts the vials into a blood counting machine that actually feeds the cells single file through a counter (just like the turn styles at the ball game).

This little magic machine records all the data and in less than a minute prints out the CBC results. Because the platelet count is low they have to manually count them for verification. They put a dab on a slide and a tech counts the number of platelet cells in a sample and then extrapolates the result to confirm the results provided by the machine. That's it for the lab.

I return to the waiting room that is by now crowded with a number of others. The HOACNY is in a six-story glass building that looks like a typical medical arts building. The fourth floor house HOACNY and there are about ten doctors in There are two different practices with about fifty or more staff members. This center includes a large waiting room, several "pods" where the administrators keep computers up to date with medical records, appointments. Etc.

There is also a large clinical area for the delivery of chemotherapy and other meds. There are fifteen stations (actually just those all too familiar ugly recliners – doctors must get a deal on those things) all occupied by patients receiving chemotherapy.

The wait time is usually not too long, and I amuse myself by picking out the veterans vs. the newcomers. The newcomers do more talking and have worried looks on their faces. You can usually spot the patient vs. a loved one by the yellow color. The veterans usually sit quietly waiting their turn. I tried to engage a few in conversations early on, but the watchword seems to be that everyone suffers in silence.

I know from observation and keeping my ears open that the group unusually includes people suffering with everything from leukemia to final stage stomach cancer. I provided taxi service for a lady from church with stage IV (that's the worst) stomach cancer for a while. She was in pretty rough shape with a continual morphine patch to alleviate her pain. She was constantly nauseous and just getting through the day was an effort. She died in late February. Makes me count my blessings!

When it is my turn to see the doctor (or more often Nurse Klinger, my advocate general), I am ushered back by a nurse who does the vitals check.

"Any pain or nausea today Mr. Lande?" "Bleeding or abnormal bruising?"
And so on it goes.
I have the answers memorized.
"No, No, No, No until they ask about the neuropathy.
"Yes, it's still there but getting better.

The nurse then takes blood pressure; temperature, pulse and I wait to see the doctor or the nurse practitioner.

When Jeff the Elder or Kathy arrives, we chat briefly about my status, they listen to my heart and we wait for the "counts" to arrive. After the first few visits, the appointments are all about the counts. If platelets or hematocrits are low, we schedule a visit to the Home Tonight center. Otherwise, I am sent home to await the next visit. Early on, I was seeing them at least once per week and by the time this book was finished; I was up to six weeks between visits.

Kathy fills out a Xeroxed form with my orders. I require irradiated, Leukopore, CMV negative blood products, which I expect, is pretty standard. They are very careful with blood products these days to avoid passing along diseases such as AIDS and Hepatitis.

CMV, Cytomegalovirus is found universally throughout all geographic locations and socioeconomic groups, and infects between 50% and 85% of adults in the United States by 40 years of age. CMV is also the virus most frequently transmitted to a developing child before birth.

For most healthy persons who acquire CMV after birth there are few symptoms and no long-term health consequences. Some persons with symptoms experience a mononucleosis-like syndrome with prolonged fever, and a mild hepatitis. Once a person becomes infected, the virus remains alive, but usually dormant within that person's body for life. Recurrent disease rarely occurs unless the person's immune system is suppressed due to therapeutic drugs or disease. Therefore, for the vast majority of people, CMV infection is not a serious problem.

However, CMV infection is important to certain high-risk groups. Major areas of concern are (1) the risk of infection to the unborn baby during pregnancy, (2) the risk of infection to people who work with children, and

(3) The risk of infection to the immunocompromised person (like AA patients), such as organ transplant recipients and persons infected with human immunodeficiency virus (HIV).

A Typical Home Tonight Visit

My appointment with Community General Hospital Home Tonight Center (CGHHTC – what can I say, I grew up in the computer industry where everything had an acronym) is usually scheduled for the next day unless I am really low (under ten on platelets or under twenty-five on hematocrits); then the transfusion is scheduled for the same day as quickly as they can take me. It is a short ten-minute drive from HOACY to CGH and I now drive myself. For the first six months or so, I could not be trusted to drive myself, so had to inconvenience family and friends.

Upon arriving at the HTC, I am usually "fast tracked" and the admission procedure does not take long at all. Every once in a while (usually at the worst times like before holidays) the normal staff is not working and the admission process can take an hour or longer. I explain that I am a regular and don't need to do all this stuff, but they don't want to hear it. They have to follow the rules and get me into their little computers.

Anyway, when I arrive at the actual HTC, "my girls", the Home Tonight team, usually greet me with smiles and cheers. They are all so friendly and upbeat, it makes the time go by faster. They all know me by name and we chat about families etc. Most of them know Sue from her days at CGH so I think I get a little more attention than the average Joe, but maybe not – everyone seems to be treated very well.

They quickly get me set up in a small cubicle designed specifically for transfusions and while the RN on duty gets the meds ordered, the LPN gets the room set up with IV pole, TV remote control (I turn on the TV with no volume to watch CNN for stock activity), pillow, blanket and a cup of coffee (this is one of the few times I indulge, but let that be our little secret).

The attending nurse checks my pulse, temperature and blood pressure every fifteen to thirty minutes. This is normally just a precaution, but there have been a few times that things have gone wrong, so I don't mind the interruption from my naps. Yes, I have learned how to nap in those ugly recliners – actually HTC has some new more attractive ones, but the mechanism and length (way too short for my 6' 3") are the same as always.

Within a few minutes, I was both flushed and connected via whatever type of catheter present or now, since the catheters are history, they need to start an IV. This is normally a simple procedure, but because I have been poke so many times, my veins are all scarred so it can get messy at times. There have been times that three or four different people had to try. They had to hot-pack my arms and do all kinds of silly things in an effort to bring my veins to the surface.

Once the IV is in place, I take my premeds (Tylenol, Benadryl and Hydrocortisone shot); wait fifteen minutes and then the blood products are hung on the pole. The platelets are pink and the blood is bright red. Both products are in little plastic bags connected via tubing to the IV in my arm. The whole delivery process is normally painless unless I have a reaction. The reaction, in my case, starts with a little itching by my mouth and then spread to my trunk. I have learned from experience to let them know right away when this starts. They stop the flow and give me more meds. If this does not happen quickly enough, I turn all red, my body is covered with hives and it is a miserable couple of hours. There have been a few times, where they gave me something strong enough to completely knock me out and we actually skipped the delivery. They advise the Red Cross to never, ever match me up with that donor (anonymous number) again and I return the next day to try again.

Chapter 11

ALG Number Two

Will it Work this Time?

On May 18, 2001, 118 days after receiving the first round of the ALG rabbit serum it was decided that we would try again. I had also been taking steroids, folic acid, Diflucan, and a whole host of other drugs that supposedly would either help the ALG work or prevent something bad from happening to me while my immune system was decreased.

The worst medication by far was that beauty called Cyclosporine. It is the worst tasting monster of a pill that I took eight does of every day. They tasted like old socks and the pills were as big around as the tip of my little finger. OK, not quite that big, but they felt that big going down

Cyclosporine is the recommended medication for trying to suppress the immune system. It apparently was not working in my case as my counts continued to stay well below normal.

So, during my monthly visit to Strong Memorial it was decided that we would try ATG or the Horse Serum treatment in the next 1-3 weeks. I'm packing my bags. Oh goodie - Hospital Food and no sleep again!

On May 28th, I was again admitted to Strong for immunosuppressive therapy. This time I was admitted to the correct floor and the preliminary work went smoothly. I was tested for any possible reaction to the ATG horse serum and apparently was going to be okay.

Apparently proved to be the operative word in that sentence! I began my first dose at 5:00 and immediately had a severe hives reaction. They decided to wait for morning and try again. No dice! My worst reaction to date convinced them that horses and I definitely do not get along. (I could have told them that based on my experience with Art and Dot's horses, but oh, well, what I know.

They had even pre-medicated me with a huge (750 MG) dose of Solumedrol (a strong antihistamine), but within only an hour of treatment it was decided that we would revert back to the ALG rabbit serum.

I was told to rest for the remainder of the day while they brewed some up for me. Who in the world ever came up with strategy anyways? Rabbit serum? Horse serum? Sounds like something the wicked witch of the east would conjure up.

The next day they started me on the ALG at a very slow rate (55 CC's per hour over ten hours and finally everything went well. I was pre-medicated with 750 Mg of Solumedrol Steroid and also made note of all the other meds I was consuming. They included:

Diflucan pill, which is an –"Anti-Fungal", designed to prevent fungal infections,

Tylenol – as a Pain Prophylactic,

Cyclosporine – the Immunosuppressant so fondly described earlier,

Magnesium – to keep magnesium levels at the necessary level (magnesium is a very important element that is often overlooked according to Sue and Dr. Rogers).

Sue did some research into magnesium and learned that magnesium is present in over 300 different enzymes in the body and that nearly every American is deficient in magnesium. It is rarely tested for yet when a person becomes seriously ill, it is one of the first things a knowledgeable doctor will prescribe.

Magnesium deficiency can be part of or the sole cause of many problems from relentless back pain, unwarranted depression, chronic fatigue, angina, hypertension, high cholesterol, nightmares, cystitis, asthma, migraines, spastic colon, leg cramps and even sudden death.

She also learned that if the body is low in magnesium it is likely low in the other trace elements of zinc, boron, copper and others. If this is true, then it is necessary to supplement all the trace elements because the body needs to the others to effectively use magnesium.

Cymedadine –an Antihistamine to prevent hives and other allergic reactions to the other medications.

Prilosec - an Anti-Nausea drug.

The next morning (May 31) my platelet counts were dangerously low (6,000) so I received platelets at 9:00. The routine of having my blood drawn at least twice each day would have been much less desirable had it not been for my friend Bernie the Hick Man!

Now that the Oh My God experience was in the distant past, the Hick Man and I had become fast friends. I could not even count the number of IV pokes I would have endured without this old pal!

The remainder of the ALG Rabbit treatments went off without a hitch except for the lack of sleep. They woke me every morning at the ungodly hour (to everyone except my buddy Jack) who arises every morning at that hour) of 4:30 A.M. to do the Dracula thing and take some of my precious blood.

Based on the latest analysis, they added potassium in the form of a beauty called K-Dur to my daily menu. This is another real beast – Actually bigger than the Cyclosporine and even more difficult to take.

My energy level was at an all-time low. It was difficult to even get out of bed but I forced myself to get up and move as much as possible. I had heard too many horror stories of people dying from pneumonia in the hospital due to fluids settling in the lungs. I was not about to be one of those statistics.

Counts on June 1st were as follows:

White Blood Cells 7.6 and okay thanks to GSF a temporary booster or growth factor

Red Blood Cells 2.9 Low

Hematocrits 27% (Low)

Platelets 17,000 (Low Low)

By June 3, they had edged up enough to allow for discharge. Behind the scenes, the docs were fighting with Sue's insurance company to allow me to stay longer, but they would have nothing of it. They did not want a repeat of last time where I was hospitalized for nearly a month. Who cares if he develops serum sickness on the way home, get him out of there!

I settled back into the routine of having my counts checked every week, receiving home health care and weekly/bi-weekly transfusions. For the first time in my life I had real insomnia. I had nightmares and had to take Ambien to help me sleep. It left me feeling drugged in the morning, but it was the only thing that would help me sleep.

I occasionally experienced some debilitating diarrhea apparently from the Prilosec because when I dropped, the diarrhea went away. The side effects warnings provided by the pharmacist now became mandatory reading for me.

I was also now the proud owner (actually just being borrowed) of my very own IV Pole for daily use in my own home. It occupies a nice spot in the corner of the bedroom and is used for the daily administration of Desferol in an effort to remove the excess iron from my body.

I really don't know why, but my Desferol was delivered via IV for several months before it was suggested that I switch to a "subcutaneous pump." I think I misunderstood what this thing was and requested the IV strategy.

Anyway for several months the chelator was delivered like any other IV med every day at home. Shelly the Bubbly One from the home care agency helped get me set up again and wished me well.

Again, after several months and actually when they pulled my last attempt at a catheter or PICC line, I was switched to the pump. This pump is very slick. It is about the size of a palmtop computer (so what else would I compare it to?) and comes complete with a little cassette full of the solutions.

You simply poke a very small needle into your belly (yes I have a big enough one), start it running and go to sleep. Nine hours later, you disconnect and you are done. Sure beats the IV routine. It is much more portable than a pole and you don't have to worry about flushing or any other plumbing.

Here are my notes from one of Shelly the Bubbly One's earlier visit in helping to set up the IV version:

1. Flush ports with 5cc of saline
2. Turn on the pump – (top left)
3. Load tubing into clamp
4. Open lever
5. Push tubing into OCC
6. Open clamp
7. Set rate at 100

Now this sounds very much like what the nurses do in the hospital and if you have ever been a visitor to one of those establishments, you know how often the nurses (with a heck of a lot more experience than yours truly) have to play around to get it working right, then you appreciate me doing the same with my little pump at home.

Sounded simple enough, but at least half the time, the pump would beep at me that it had air in the line and the whole routine would have to be reset. A large pain!

Following about 2-3 hours of solution, then disconnect, flush with saline and heparin and ok now you can put the pole back in its place in the corner.

I had a talk with Lucy yesterday and she registered concern that my White Blood Cell counts are not stabilizing and they are not sure what to do about it. The GSF growth factor shots are only temporary boosters and will not work it they are used too often. Without the White Blood Cells, I will be unable to resist even a basic common cold.

I had been corresponding online with Mindy by now and asked Lucy if Cytoxan might be an option for me. She promised to check into it and I also did my own research.

Cytoxan is another experimental drug that has been used successfully by Dr. Brodsky at Johns Hopkins to place several AA types into a durable remission. The downside is that apparently Dr. Young at National Institute of Health had also tested the drug with disastrous results.

Supposedly it killed 3 people in 3 months, so there is now a raging debate going on between the two teams. Brodsky claims they did not administer it properly and Young claims it is far too dangerous and needs further testing. What's a Bubba to do? My life is on the line and so far nothing appears to be working!

Most of June and July included weekly treks to Rochester and Strong Memorial for shots and CBC's. Good news was that platelets held at 14,000 so have held for 12 days - longest on record - cautious optimism. Shots included Neuprin, Epogin and GSF all designed to "boost" blood cell production.

I was also administered something called "TPA" to help loosen clogged port and was advised to increase my port flushing routine to twice a day. Port flushing? What am I, a plumber? Yes, it seems that the Hick Man can easily become clogged so I must "push" a saline cleansing agent to keep them open.

In the beginning, the nurses did this for me, but I am now more self-sufficient and can flush with the best of them. I am warned that proper technique (wear gloves, wash hands, do not breath on my site) is critical as even the slightest infection could kill me.

The Hick Man is directly connected to my heart and Bernie can deliver germs very quickly. I also have to clean the "site" where the catheter enters my chest every day and again must use very careful technique. A good part of my day is absorbed in cleaning and flushing and taking meds.

When time was available, I tried to research ways to get myself better, but must admit it had by now become very discouraging. Since AA is not really on anybody's radar screen, there is not much going on. BMT, ATG, ALG, Cyclosporine and Cytoxan are about it for options and none of them appeared to be working or viable for me.

Chapter 12

The Bargaining Begins

The Emotional Aspects

By this time, I was past the anger and denial stages and was into bargaining. I would strike bargains with everyone I met. God, my wife, doctors, nurses - everywhere I went, life was barter. I'll take that pill if you leave me alone for a while. If I am really good, can I get out of the hospital now? God - let me live long enough to see Melissa married and I'll promise to be good. I'll go to church and I'll even sing in the choir. I did, she did, and I do.

The five official, psychiatrist endorsed, phases of dealing with death are Anger, Denial, Bargaining, Depression and Acceptance. My reactions were not in such a neat order, and I still go in and out of all of them on a regular basis. I can honestly say that I have now faced death and am better for it.

It helped me to appreciate what I have and to spend more time on the truly important things we have while here on earth. As Father Walsh, the pastor who married Sue and I said: "I shall not pass this way again, any kindness I may do, let me do it now, for I shall not pass this way again."

I am still too self-centered to ever be a Father Walsh, but I work much harder at being kinder and more tolerant towards others. I spend more time listening to my children and just being with my wife. I sing in the choir and enjoy the fellowship of others in the church. I watch the snowfall, I listen to the wind and I cradle my wife at night. When I was alone at night in my hospital bed I began to chronicle my life and realized what a waste much of it had been. I now have a new chance and I am doing my best to give back.

The Anger phase was and has been short lived for me. My anger was mostly about what I would leave behind rather than a concern for myself. Since losing my job with Digital and starting the business, and now with my illness our financial position had gotten progressively worse. At one time, I figured we were in the top 5% of the socio-economic scale and we were now heading for the bottom 25%. I did not want to leave my wife in that position.

Luckily, we have been able to downsize and rescale our situation so that I can rest better at night, but it took some very drastic measures in a relatively short time frame. I will admit that I also had feelings of anger towards God who seemed to be dumping on us once again but after several sessions with our new pastor I began to feel less anger and more comfort.

Funny some of the things you remember, but one that really sticks out for me is my very first "personal" communion service. Pastor Derron visited me in my house and brought along the bread and wine for a personal blessing. It made me cry!

Later, while I was in the hospital he offered it again and I shared it with my sister-in-law Kathie who has been one of my most steadfast supporters during this ordeal. It was a very comforting moment and I guess a form of accepting my own eventual death. I actually felt that way several times and it was a very strange feeling knowing that I may not see another sunrise. I fought sleep several times fearing that I would not wake up.

Most of my current anger is directed at the IRS for wanting me to pay taxes on an IRA hardship withdrawal and POMCO ("The largest self-insurance company in New York State") for not paying my medical bills.

My question to the IRS is this: "When I am dead, will you come after my wife to pay this bill?" Knowing them, I am quite confident they will not let this sleeping dog lie, so in addition to the pain of losing me, she will have to deal with the relentless pursuit of the tax collectors.

Denial was and is a much easier stage for me. I have always been very self-reliant and refuse to accept the fact that anything can stop me from getting what I want. I had been successful in my career, been a very competitive athlete and built two houses with my own bare hands. I still have a hard time believing that anything can stop me.

Then I look at my hands - Even today, after two years of battling AA, they are yellow and washed out. And I visit the doctor to learn that my "counts" are still far from normal. A "chronic, often fatal blood disease" is something that happens to other people. I don't do hospitals. The smell alone nauseates me.

I have now been in one kind of hospital or another (as a patient for the first time in over 40 years) for nearly 300 days in the past two years. I once calculated that I spent over 200 of the 365 days in 2001 in a doctor's office, hospital or treatment center. Even through all this, I am sure that I am the exception to the rule and can make myself better. I will not die young. I have too many things yet to do. Some may call it denial; I call it Self Preservation.

Depression is the one that surprised me. I can't ever remember feeling really depressed for one moment in my life prior to the illness. I used to consider it a sign of weakness. Yet here I was actually feeling sorry for myself, wallowing in self-pity even to a point that my good friend Jack had to give me a verbal kick in the pants.

I don't remember the exact words any more, but it was after a fairly long time of listening to me moan and groan when he spoke from the heart.

He said: "I have been here for you and will continue to be here for you, but there is one thing I will not do, I will not listen to you cry about your situation." Jack had seen and experienced more by the time he was twenty-two years old than I will experience in my entire life. He was a First Lieutenant in Vietnam and held many a dying man in his arms. It reminds me of the movie "Rules of Engagement" when asked what the average life expectancy of a First Lieutenant was in Vietnam - The response was "Thirty Minutes".

Now, whenever I get feeling sorry for myself, I think of Jack and all the others who gave their youth to a war nobody wanted - sleeping on the ground in a jungle thousands of miles from home. I did my time during that era but was always safe in my bed at night. I consider it a tragedy that the many young men and women who gave their youth and lives to that undeclared war returned to an ungrateful nation.

I am honored to have several very good friends who have stuck by me throughout this ordeal and I am happy to put Jack and Liz at the very top next to Sue and Kathie. Jack and his wife Liz dropped everything to be at my bedside in the emergency room. It was Jack's birthday and they were dressed to the nines ready for a night on the town.

Instead, they spent hours offering support to Sue and Melissa and a couple of nights later showed up with a take-out dinner from our favorite restaurant, the Dinosaur Bar-B-Que" The best little Honky Tonk Blues Joint in the world.

IRS Update and a good outlet for my anger:

I just received letter number two from the IRS stating that we owe them $9,000 for an early withdrawal from my IRA that was essentially used to pay the doctor bills our insurance company would not cover. Just when I was beginning to see the light, I get hit with this. Incredible!

I have paid more taxes in my life than most people earn and now when I am in trouble they want to take a sucker punch? After the first letter, I sent off a lengthy letter explaining my circumstances and their response basically ignored my letter and said Pay up, even if we have to deduct it from your disability check - what am I missing here? One branch of government is helping me to stay alive and now a different branch wants the money back. I think I'll write a book.

Chapter 13

Your New Life

The Saga Continues

It is now July of 2001 and my life is focused almost entirely on this stupid illness. I spent almost every day this past week either in the CGH Home Tonight or a Doctor's office of one kind or another.

Monday I was at Kirshner and the HOACNY for a CBC. Platelets were 5000 so I spent a good part of Tuesday getting platelets. The actual procedure of getting the platelets can take as little as fifteen to twenty minutes, for most people, but because of all my reactions, it ends up taking well over two hours for the whole process and then there is the check in time, waiting afterwards to make sure I am ok and the transportation time. It pretty much consumes the day.

Wednesday was the Fourth of July so I got a day off. Thursday I am back to HOACNY for check of hematocrits as they were close on Monday. Yep, they are down to 23,000 so guess what? Yep, Friday is back to CGH and home tonight. Judy, the admission receptionists sees me coming and has everything waiting for me in advance now I am such a regular.

I arrive at 11:00 AM and finally get back home at 7:30 PM. The following Monday, platelets are again at 5,000 and we start all over again. Platelets only last six or seven days so I guess this is going to be my life for a while. Today's experience is even worse however because I again have a serious reaction. My whole body turns in to one big hive. I have huge welts all over my body and the itching is unbearable. They give me twice as much Benadryl as usual and two hydrocortisone shots but the rash persists so they give up and send me home with NO PLATELETS! We will try again tomorrow. Tuesday goes Ok and after eight days of almost constant doctoring I finally get a couple days of rest. This is almost as bad as being in the hospital. I virtually have no life! I felt pretty lousy all week. Even a short walk wiped me out. I am getting progressively weaker and can't exercise to keep up my strength. Is this what my life is going to be like?

July 12, 2001 – Journal Entry:

Good News Day!

I received some very exciting news today after a thorough conversation with my care team at Strong Memorial Hospital in Rochester, NY. They are recommending me for an Unrelated Matched Donor (MUD) Bone Marrow Transplant preceded by a T Cell depletion strategy that substantially reduces the risk of Graft vs. Host Disease (GVHD).

My good friend Ray spent the whole day with me in Rochester where I had a CBC, cultures, Pentamidine (anti-parasitic), the usual pre meds and Platelets. I also had my three shots for growth stimulation Neupogen, Epogen and GSF. I was very tired afterwards but excited about the potential transplant.

At least we are going to try something rather than continue this seemingly endless round of transfusions and growth shots. Nothing seems to be doing any good so I guess the transplant is a necessary evil. I mention to them that I will be attending the AA/MDS Patient Conference in St. Louis so the procedure is tentatively scheduled for September 17th in Rochester.

Chapter 14

AA/MDS Conference

St. Louis Trip Report

Although the decision to go forward with the transplant feels ok, I am still somewhat reluctant and Sue shares with me that she is very concerned about this approach. We agree to discuss it more fully while on our trip.

I had been in contact with the Aplastic Anemia and MDS Foundation early on and Marilyn Baker, the Executive Director invited me to attend the annual patient conference. I initially didn't see that it would be very helpful but now after two failed ATG attempts and my virtual dependency on transfusions I was becoming desperate.

I hoped that the conference would provide some answers.

Following the

A Trip to St. Louis & Beyond

Sue, Melissa and I decided to attend the annual AA-MDS patient conference in St Louis even though I was very concerned about air travel (breathing others people's germs for several hours in a closed environment is not healthy for children and other sensitive beings).

Coincidentally, my nephew was to be married around the same time in Iowa so we decided to take advantage of the opportunity and see relatives that we had not seen in many years. Sue had sent out word that I was not well so several family members stayed an extra day to spend time with us. It was great to see everyone although I would have preferred different circumstances.

After two or three days with my sister Martha, brother Greg and other family members I was pretty well wiped out. At my request, Rochester had pre-arranged a blood and platelet transfusion for me in Des Moines and that gave me enough energy to do the conference that had been the original reason for the trip.

The conference was held at a Marriot Hotel near the airport and we arrived Friday afternoon. The main conference was scheduled for Saturday, but there were additional activities on Friday evening and Sunday.

Friday was a bit of a disappointment as there was not really much going on but I remained optimistic about Saturday. We met a few other patients but most of them appeared to be MDS types rather than AA and we had a hard time linking up with people who were in the same situation as we were.

There were, however a couple of reasonably good presentations. Probably the best one for me was by a patient named David Biro who was also an M.D. although his presence at the seminar was in his role as a patient. He talked candidly about his experience and sold his book "One Hundred Days" following his presentation. I bought the book and looked forward to reading it on the way home.

From a presentation entitled "Non Transplant Treatments for AA and PNH" by Dr. Lucio Luzzatto, M.D., the Scientific Director IST, Genoa, Italy and the keynote speaker we learned that the preferred treatment for Bone Marrow Failure is still a Bone Marrow Transplant, but when there are high risks or extenuating circumstances, then one must consider alternatives.

The currently most popular alternative is ATG, a very powerful immunosuppressant and Cyclosporine.

According to Dr. Luzzatto, this combination is successful approximately 70% of the time but does not often result in a durable cure. The supportive treatment options include Red Cell Transfusions, Platelet Transfusions, Growth Factor Shots and Prophylactic Antibiotics. Unfortunately the only reliable current treatment for "hemolysis" is to replace the blood. It is humbling, but true that after all these years - there is no other treatment.

Management Options:

- Radical - BMT/Self-Care
- Softer Options - Immunosuppression
- Live With It - Supportive Treatment

The common denominator of AA, MDS, and PNH is Bone Marrow Failure. AA & PNH are very closely related. He went on to describe more about his obvious predilection in something called PNH but it held little interest for me. PNH or Paroxysmal Nocturnal Hemoglobinuria occurs because of a somatic mutation (it is not hereditary), in any cell of the body it occurs in the pig a gene of the X chromosome.

The PigA chromosome creates a molecule that anchors proteins to the membrane. The fundamental problem with PNH is that this anchor is not properly produced, and on and on he went on something about which I could not have cared less!

We then had another talk from a Dr. Richard Champlin from the Houston Medical Center on Transplants for Aplastic Anemia. The Houston Center is one of the top two or three transplant centers in the country. The others are the Fred Hutchins Center in Seattle, the Dana Farber Institute in Boston and the Johns Hopkins Center in Philadelphia.

I had considered the possibility of transferring to one of these centers but had become comfortable with the people in Rochester and Syracuse and knew that they consulted with the other centers on a regular basis.

I was expecting a little more than Dr. Champlin provided, but I guess I must have been better informed than others in the audience.

He explained that Aplastic Anemia is a Stem Cell Disease –and results from a primary failure of or injury to the bone marrow. MDS, on the other hand, is a clonal proliferation of defective hematopoietic cells. AML or Adult Myeloid Leukemia is a clonal proliferation of cancerous hematopoietic cells in other parts of the body. Extended AML can result in MDS or Leukemia.

He reiterated how AA results from "a primary failure of the bone marrow to produce a number of blood cells."

He went on to say how AA is most often discovered when a patient presents with Pancytopenia (low blood cell counts) and a hypo cellular marrow. The pathophysiology indicates that there has been an injury to the stem cells that are responsible for producing all types of blood cells.

The cells are damaged as pluripotent stem cells (precursors to blood cells) before they are even fully developed and the immune system destroys them before they are allowed into the blood stream.

He then discussed the various transplant and other treatment options that were available including both the generally accepted ones and the ones still considered to be experimental. He indicated that Cytoxan was still considered to be very high risk by most centers. –

Hopkins and Dr. Brodsky say that has been very successful but Houston and most other center and especially Dr. Young of the National Institute of Health are opposed to the protocol. –

According to Dr. Champlin, the predominant strategy right now is to make Bone Marrow Transplants less risky by:
1. Reducing the level of radiation
2. Decreasing the likelihood of graft
3. Depleting the T Cells and limiting the immune response

There were a few other presentations that for the most part did not apply to us. Perhaps the most revealing part of the whole exercise came when we actually met some people who had been through BMT's.

It was very frightening to see what they looked like. Many had lost a hip or walked with a limp. Several who had been through it most recently had no hair and were very gaunt looking. It was one thing to read about side effects, it was an entirely different experience to actually see and talk to the people!

Sue said, "This is what I have been trying to tell you, Bubba. It will not be a pleasant experience and you very likely might die or be crippled for life if you go through with what you are considering."

I must admit that the trip to St. Louis really had me second- guessing my decision to do the transplant. To make matters worse, I completely ran out of gas on Sunday and knew that I would be back on the transfusion routine when we returned to New York.

Unfortunately, we left the Midwest with more questions than answers and I was now for the first time actually frightened by what might happen next.

Chapter 15
Now What Are My Options?

Where from Here?

I talked to many people at the conference about transplant and read the book "One Hundred Days" by Dr. David Biro on the plane trip home. I am quite sure that he was painting his story as a success but it scared the heck out of me.

He described the entire experience including a time when he was so weak that he lost consciousness and fell in the shower. He was obviously so weak at times and his immune system was so compromised that he could have easily died from the experience.

July 12th, 2001

The good news is that I have now lived beyond the original six months Jeff the Elder gave me. The bad news is that I am getting progressively weaker and do not seem to have very many viable treatment options remaining.

Sue, Melissa and I are meeting with Jeff the Younger and his faithful companions, Sharon and Lucy. It is by now apparent that ATG is not going to work for me and the question is where do we go from here?

My alternatives are:

1.	A Full Bone Marrow Transplant - High Risk

2. Cytoxan - Mixed Results
3. Mini Transplant - Fludarapine Melapine
4. Transplant with T Cell Depletion -HMO IV

We discuss how the best alternative is the one with lowest risk of GVHD because it is GVHD that causes all the problems we witnessed in St. Louis.

I really don't know what to do now. If I stay with the ATG/Cyclosporine and nothing happens I may be opting out of the transplant alternative whether I want to or not. If I go for the transplant I either die or go through hell with lots of serious side effects as a result.

I ask Jeff the Younger to look into the Hopkins Cytoxan program Even though he and nearly everyone associated with the AA Foundation is very much against it; I have been talking online with Mindy. She is actual survivor of the program and swears by it. She says that NIH is against it because they did not administer the program properly and rather than admit their mistake they claim the process itself is faulty.

Jeff the Younger reluctantly agrees and says we will talk further during our next visit. He does indeed make contact with Dr. Brodsky and they discuss my situation directly. It turns out that one of the reasons the NIH test had failed is that they worked with patients who had previously been on Cyclosporine and since that fit my situation the Cytoxan treatment could not be attempted until I had been completely off the Cyclosporine and all other immune- suppressants for at least six months.

The Rochester BMT team wants to keep me on the Cyclosporine for a bit longer and see if it might work.

Oh great, I think, it doesn't work anyway and now I have to decide whether I want to continue taking that dreadful stuff or drop it altogether and opt for the experimental drug treatment that could just kill me outright. I did not much like my choices.

After much discussion, we finally agreed to give the second ALG and Cyclosporine a little longer. But I must admit I was not at all hopeful.

Meanwhile, Sue had continued to pursue the alternative treatments mentioned to her by Dr. Sherry Rogers, her Environmental Illness Doctor. While I was debating the least of several evils, she tried to make an appointment to discuss my situation with Dr. Rogers.

Unfortunately Dr. Rogers was no longer taking on new patients but they did talk on the phone and she said, "If it were my husband, he would be on the next plane to Texas. There is an Environment Health Center there that I went to when I had given up all hope. It worked for me and I encourage you to contact them immediately."

On August 18, 2001 I decided that the ATG/Cyclosporine was officially a failed treatment protocol for me and threw all my drugs in the trash.

Chapter 16

Trip to Dallas

The EHCD

"The doctor of the future will give no medicine, but will interest his patients in the care of the human frame, in diet, and in the cause and prevention of disease."

--Thomas Edison

This chapter in our lives started with a departure from the nearly defunct Syracuse International Airport. When I was the DEC (Digital Equipment Corporation) Account Manager for what was left of Carrier Corporation this little airport was a bustle of activity.

There were six or seven flights per day to most cities in the Northeast including Boston, my usual destination. I was on a project team that required me to attend a bi-weekly meeting in Marlboro, Mass. I would leave my house about 6:30 am, fly to Logan, catch a Digital helicopter shuttle and begin my meeting by 10:00. It was a magnificent feeling to fly over the Charles River and all the traffic. That was the fun part.

Too often, my meetings would end on Friday afternoon and I would scramble to catch a flight before bad weather set in. Unfortunately, I spent many a wintry Friday night stranded at Logan airport hoping to get to Syracuse via any route possible.

* * * * *

In 2001, The Syracuse airport was empty most of the day and the flight load would hardly raise an eyebrow. What did raise a few eyebrows was our attire. I had been advised to avoid plane travel due to the germs floating around in airports and especially in the confined quarters of the airplane itself where the germs of every patient are circulated and then re-circulated for all passengers to enjoy.

So, to keep me safe from all those germs, my sister-in-law Kathie provided us with the cutest imitation of a Donald Duck mask I had ever seen. Pink in color these ugly ducklings were designed to protect "preemies" from the nasty germs of the world into which they had recently been born. Kathie has been a neonatal nurse at one of Syracuse's remaining "real" hospitals for as long as I have known her, which is about thirty years.

Kathie and Sue had been trail bosses back at Scenic Valley Riding Stables and it is there that I first met her and my brother-in-law Laverne Doctor. Vern has been a trusted friend for many years and would have laughed himself silly had he seen the little group of ugly ducklings making their way through the Hancock Terminal.

Hancock Field is also home to the "Boys of Syracuse" one of the first battle groups to be scrambled after the attack on the World Trade Center. Our trip began on July 9, 2001. Phase one continued until that fateful day in September. My situation paled in comparison, but at this point we did not know what lay ahead. I had by now either been through or seriously investigated all the conventional treatments for Aplastic Anemia.

With an incredible amount of research behind us, we were now trekking through the Syracuse airport like little lost ducklings on our way to Dallas, Texas for what felt like our last hope. As Sue says, we would never get away with wearing these masks post 9/11, but for this trip we were just silly looking novelties.

In early August of 2001 I stopped all medications and began the "grains, greens and beans" macrobiotic diet prescribed by Dr. Rogers. Sue has been a patient of Dr. Sherry Rogers, an Environmental Allergist MD here in Syracuse.

After hearing of my symptoms, Dr. Rogers recommended that I immediately contact Dr. William Re at the Environmental Health Center in Dallas, TX. I was extremely skeptical about the approach, but after much cajoling from Sue, I finally decided to make the trip to Dallas.

* * * * *

On August 18, Sue and I arrived in Dallas courtesy of our good friend Liz and United Airlines. Liz had secured some buddy passes for us and we were able to move from interest to action in the matter of a few hours.

On August 20 we had our first meeting with Dr. Rea. His clinic was not at all what I had pictured. I envisioned sort of an upscale spa like atmosphere in a suburban setting. Instead it was on the second floor of a very unassuming medical building not too far from downtown Dallas.

After a bit of confusion with the outer office staff we were finally ushered into a small sparsely appointed exam room. Dr. Rea is a scholarly looking older gentleman; he appears to be in his mid to late 70's and walks with a severe limp. He pulled up one of those little stools docs like to use and after only a few minutes, I decided that he was someone I could trust.

He had obviously read some of the notes we forwarded (we sent letters from Dr. Kirshner and Dr. Lancet's office with some chart information) He asked about Dr. Rogers and he and Sue chatted politely for a few minutes.

He then asked me about how I had been progressing with the illness and what meds I had been taking. He then asked me to do the strangest thing. He essentially had me take a sobriety test in his office. He asked me to try and stand on one leg.

"No problem", I thought as I had always had good athletic balance. I gave it a try and to my amazement, was unable to balance for even a few seconds. Next, he asked me to walk heal to toe in a straight line. I again failed miserably!

It was as though I was intoxicated. He gently explained, as no doubt he has done hundreds of other times that indeed I was toxic. My body was loaded with all sorts of toxic drugs, pesticides and chemicals and as a result, my brain was not functioning properly. The fundamental message appeared to be that my immune system was out of whack and probably had been for many years.

We discussed my concern that according to everything I have read, an inability to produce megakaryocytes (listen to me would you!) could be a showstopper. He said, "I no longer believer in showstoppers. I have seen too many successes after others have given up hope." - I think I'm going to like this guy!

He went on to say, "We would leave no stone unturned until we find something we can work on and we will get to the bottom of this." He also warned that it can be a very tedious process and we are not to expect any silver bullets.

He gave us a small ray of hope but was careful to tell us that there would be no miracles. I will go through a battery of tests before he would make any recommendations and whatever we do, it is going to take time and a dedicated effort on my part.

He closed by saying, "Let's give this a whirl and see how it goes." Not exactly the most encouraging news I had heard lately, but possibly the most honest!

Within a few short days, the first "alternative" approach was officially in process. I had dramatically changed my environment and my eating habits. Sue and I were living in a chemically safe apartment that was very sparsely furnished, had no carpets, had a filtered air system and much to my chagrin; I could already actually feel a difference.

We were on a very restrictive rotational diet designed to isolate foods to which I may be allergic. We had four different plans that were rotated over four days. For example, on day one, I would eat bananas and almonds for breakfast; lentil beans, carrots and onions for lunch; and chicken, green beans and sweet potatoes for dinner. This part was the most difficult for me as I was a fast food junkie and ate lots of meat and potatoes.

The good news was that after some of the preliminary testing, Dr. Rea had agreed to take on my case. I had also some done some Internet research and learned a bit more about him. Dr. William Rea is a world-renowned practitioner of environmental medicine and is the founder of the Environment Health Center Foundation of Dallas.

The website at ehcd.com was not up to my professional standards <grin>, but was informative. Like so many other MD's who have "seen the light", he himself suffered from chemical illness and has developed a program to assist others in healing their own bodies. He is a renowned cardiac and thoracic specialist and in fact was on the team that tried to save President John Kennedy's life back in '63.

He is highly intelligent, has authored a series of four textbooks on environmental illness and has devoted his professional life in efforts to raise the awareness of how the toxins and poisons in our environment are killing us. Unfortunately because he is going against the money of the pharmaceutical industry, he has been labeled a "quack" and the medical establishment undermines many of his efforts.

I had been on my own version of a detoxification program and macrobiotic diet for two weeks before coming to Texas and have now been on the rotational diet for two weeks. I am starting to feel a little better but unfortunately still have a long ways to go and am having a real hard time accepting the necessary changes.

It would be necessary to continue on this protocol for at least another two months and be patient in looking for improvement.

Update August 28, 2001

After one month on the EHCD program, my counts remain about the same (so no harm is being done) but I do feel much better without any of the ugly side effects of Cyclosporine and other drugs. I am not yet in any position to recommend this approach to others but am using myself as a human guinea pig and will certainly let everyone know the results.

What I have done so far:

I started by dropping all meds about a month ago. I've subsequently read that this should be done slowly using a tapered strategy rather than just quitting cold turkey. Next, I went on a macrobiotic diet as recommended by Dr. Sherry Rogers (my wife's Environmental Illness MD) in her book "The Cure is in the Kitchen" (See Book List). The diet consisted of "Grains, Greens and Beans" and I also undertook the detoxification process she recommended.

I felt lousy for a while, but then better as I dropped all meat, dairy and what she calls "deadly night shades" (peppers, potatoes, cucumbers and tomatoes). The meals were dreadfully bland, but they did clear my gastrointestinal system. Then on her recommendation we came to Texas and began testing with Dr. Rea.

Let me try and describe the environment at the Environmental Health Center (ok, ok, I know):

This place is like a boot camp for the chemically sensitive. The walls and floor are virtually bare. There are no carpets, wall hangings or anything that could collect dust or give off chemical toxins. Even the furniture is steel or wood. Not very comfortable I might add.

I learn that the entire facility has been repainted using chemically safe paint and there are air cleaners in every room. No newspapers or any other printed materials are allowed in the testing or treatment areas because many of the patients are allergic to newsprint and ink.

All patients must wear only cotton clothes with no hair spray, perfumes or any offensive odors. No smoking! You are not even allowed to go outside and smoke and then return because we can smell it on your clothes. If you want to get well, you will not smoke!

The rules are strictly enforced and any offenders are immediately removed from the program. I actually saw this happen a little later on when a lady claimed she was no longer smoking but we could all smell it one her. She threw a fit and the Nurse Manager physically removed her from the building –It was quite a scene.

When we are not at the center receiving treatments, we are holed up in another aesthetically pleasing environment – the "condos." These condos are actually 1950 vintage apartments with; you guessed it, no carpets, no wall hangings and the most uncomfortable furniture you can imagine. The kitchen set is wrought iron and the living room "sofa" is a wooden park bench. That is the extent of the furniture with the exception of the bedroom.

Now the bedroom, here's a treat. There are no real mattresses, as we know them. The mattress consists of several cotton blankets wrapped by a sheet on a bed that is about five feet long. Doesn't fit my six-foot frame very well. Yes, I feel like I am back in boot camp! Mattresses are great breeding places for mites and bold and the cotton blankets can be easily laundered.

Within a very short time, we were seriously engaged in the program including the rotation diet mentioned earlier. We eat somewhat normal foods but are restricted to certain foods each meal, e.g. yesterday we had eggs and pineapple for breakfast; lettuce, walnuts and alfalfa sprouts for lunch and hamburger, potatoes and peas for dinner - no ketchup or other spices.

This is by far the most normal day of the four rotational days. Other days we have had quinoa for breakfast, spinach for lunch and salmon for dinner.

I am also undergoing many tests: being injected with minute amounts of various chemicals to determine if I am sensitive to anything (formaldehyde, lead, silver, serotonin, magnesium, etc.).

I have also had a themography to test for abnormalities in my organs. It clearly showed malfunctions in my kidney and liver. Pupillography which verified poor oxygen flow, EMF testing to see if I had problems with electro-magnetic fields, which turned out to be negative, and a three-stage urinalysis that we will see results for in a couple of weeks.

I have also had a number of blood tests that are still being evaluated. Dr. Rea said from the beginning that he was not sure if he could help or not. His honesty is refreshing but I had hoped for some results by now.

He is still very cautious and doesn't even really have a sense of when he might know if he can help or not. So far he is just gathering information and will continue to do so for at least a couple of weeks if not longer.

He did have me start on a physical therapy regimen yesterday that includes some light exercise, a sauna and a massage. This is designed to help rid my body of toxins that have been building up over many years.

August 24

I had a terrible reaction to platelet transfusion today. Must be the platelets are different in Texas? They were single donor, irradiated, Leukopore, and CMV negative and I had my normal pre-meds (Tylenol, Hydrocortisone and Benadryl) followed by a second dose but still got slammed!

I had a burning and itching rash from the bottom of my feet to the top of my head. It was by far the worst case yet and they finally gave me an Attarax that after about an hour knocked me out.

Mid-August

Sue has been my constant companion throughout the ordeal and has been an unbelievable source of support. There were many days that I did not have the strength to walk to the car and back without help. I was like an 80 year old man. No, I was worse than that – Grandpa is 80 and he doesn't need help. She planned the special meals, bought and carried the groceries, cooked the meals, kept up my spirits, chauffeured me back and forth to the center, ferried me to the hospital for transfusions and rescued me when I had the severe reaction to Texas blood.

But, it is time for her to return to work and help plan for Melissa's wedding so I will drive her to the airport tomorrow and hope that I can return to my Texas home safely.

September 2, 2001

It has now been nearly eight months since my diagnosis and I am probably more hopeful than I have been in six months. It is way too early to declare even a small victory but judging strictly on how I feel, I think this natural healing and detoxification approach has a chance.

I reached a pinnacle today in that sweat was literally pouring off my body in the sauna. I have never been one to sweat very much even while an athlete in high school so this is a new experience for me.

The veteran patients here say this is a big step towards ridding your body of harmful chemicals and toxins that have been building up in your digestive system and immune system for many years and it really does feel good.

I have also been testing for allergies to chemicals, molds, foods and minerals and learning what compounds with which I may be having problems. Once they establish what the testers call "end points" they will develop antigens to those substances that I will then inject on a regular basis to help my system deal with them.

In the beginning this whole approach seemed a bit far-fetched, but at least for now, it is making some sense and I am hopeful. I have been repeatedly cautioned that there are no "silver bullets" and this is potentially a long arduous process, but I have now met some people (granted not AA types) who are finding success in dealing with diseases that other MD's have given up on.

September 8, 2001 - Natural Healing Setback

Well, the platelet counts only held for two weeks but considering my previous record was 10 days, I am still somewhat hopeful. Also got another infection in my site and had a negative reaction to Desferol. Was awake most of last Friday night with fever and chills. Oh what I would give to be "normal" again. Spending almost full time in testing, sauna, exercising and talking with Doctors, Nurses and other patients. Platelet counts were 14,000 on Friday so my Saturday afternoon was spent getting a platelet transfusion (approaching 100 transplants now). Had attempted to work my upper body last week to regain some strength and then contracted the infection so am backing off a bit - Will hit it again next week. I remain cautiously optimistic but it is a lot of work to stay with this program. Oh well - Nothing ventured, nothing gained.

September 15, 2001 - Melissa & Mike Get Married

I was scheduled to fly home for the wedding on Thursday. On Tuesday, 9/11/2001 the WTC and Pentagon were attacked so all flights were cancelled. I left Dallas at 8:30 Wednesday morning; met Melanie and Fred in Tri Cities, TN at 10:30 PM, dropped off rental car and then completed trip to Syracuse. We arrived on Thursday evening and thanks to unbelievable work by Sue, Melissa, Kathy and others the wedding went off beautifully. It was a proud day for Mom and Dad to have everyone together and to witness the love shared by Mike and Melissa. Their honeymoon had to be postponed because of the terrorist attack but they spent a couple of days in the Pocono's.

September 25, 2001 - Cautious Optimism - Positive Attitude and Financial Woes

I had a CBC before leaving from Texas to Syracuse, one while I was there and one upon my return. I feel better than I have in 6 months and my time between transfusions is increasing. I am now exercising 20-30 minutes each day; my brain is clearing (can walk the straight line) and with the exception of a severe pain in my shoulder, I am able to almost function normally. I still sleep more than I used to but the time between transfusions (24+ days for blood and 13 days for platelets has me thinking positively about Dr. Rea and EHCD. Time will tell. I feel really good!

Testing continues - Had a very severe reaction to grass - no more mowing lawns for a living! Actually getting used to the rotation diet and it doesn't seem as bad anymore. Daily exercise, sauna and massage are working - I sweat more than I have in my entire life and am supposedly ridding my body of harmful toxins (you can tell by the smell!).

I miss Sue terribly. We talked last night but got into financial issues. It was very troubling. It does not appear that our insurance pay for any of this. It is costing $70 per day to stay here plus Dr. visits, vitamins, special diet, testing and now they want me to buy a sauna ($5000) and redo the new house we just moved into (or move). No carpets where I will be spending most of my time (house is wall to wall) and he wants the furnace outside of the house because of my sensitivity to natural gas. Who is going to pay for all this?

The money we raised in the golf tournament is long gone and we are now eating away at our retirement (which was already way down due to lousy investments). Sue to contact patient advocate organization. Now that I am finally making some progress health wise, the financial issues are overwhelming!

Update September 26, 2001

This strategy may work! It has been twenty-five days since my last blood transfusion and I am feeling stronger than at any time in the past six months (thirty minutes of exercise every day). There are none of the side effects associated with Cyclosporine and the other drugs.

I am faithfully (well almost) following the rotational diet, taking about 10 different vitamins and supplements every day, exercising, sauna and massage daily.

I have also done about 50 different tests and have discovered that I am allergic to milk products, beef, chicken, brewer's yeast, grass, and about 20 other compounds.

The testing process consists of injecting a small amount of each substance into the shoulder, measuring the initial site with a little "wheal card" and then rechecking it in ten minutes to see if the "wheal" has grown in size. If it grows a small amount, you are determined have a mild allergy and if it grows by a larger amount, you have a severe reaction.

I only had one serious reaction and that was to grass! My whole shoulder swelled up almost immediately. Now that may explain why I suffer with sneezing, runny nose and sinus headaches every spring when the new grass appears!

It was also recommended that I avoid milk products and beef.

Once they determine what substances can cause allergic reactions, they develop an antigen and you then give yourself antigen shots on a rotating basis. In the end, my antigen shots include:

- Foods as mentioned
- Grass and molds
- Bacteria
- CMV
- IV Nutrients
- Metals
- Natural Gas
- Orris Root (Fragrance found in everything)

I take antigen shots every day and am considering the purchase of a sauna for home. It is definitely an all-consuming program that will require major life changes but if it is going to save my life it is well worth the effort.

Dr. Rea and I discussed potential causes yesterday and are pretty much in agreement that it is a case of "Multiple Chemical Sensitivity." After being exposed to many new houses, grass (big time reaction), pesticides, etc., my immune system finally just shut down.

Now that we are moving many of the toxins via sauna and exercise, my body is responding appropriately. There is still a long ways to go, but for the first time in quite a while I am allowing myself to think beyond the next week or two.

Whilst all the allergic testing is proceeding, I am also subjected to other tests and allowed to try other regimens. The physical therapy is my favorite as I can actually feel myself getting stronger as time goes on. The first venture into physical therapy was not very promising. I walked the treadmill for about two minutes and had to stop. I then entered the low heat sauna room and lasted about ten minutes.

As I progressed to thirty minutes of fairly strenuous exercise and two forty-five minute high heat sauna sessions per day, I began to feel like there was hope again. Early on I would not sweat at all and I would marvel at the outpouring from the vets. Within a few weeks I was sweating with the best of them.

It was very refreshing to be ridding myself of toxins knowing that each day brought more energy and a clearer mind. For the first time in over a year, I was able to completely think through a though pattern. Previously my mind would just completely blank out right in the middle. I suspected I was an early candidate for Alzheimer's but then realized that it had been the toxins all along.

Besides the sauna/physical therapy, I tried the oxygen therapy but did not stay with that one very long. It involved sitting in a room by myself with a special plastic mask over my face for a full hour. The mask was attached to a rack of copper tubes and then into an oxygen tank.

I had to sit in this room by myself for an hour with nothing to but breathe. No books, no CD, just breathe! The time passed like molasses through a 5cc syringe (oh, my god, medical analogies.)

September 28 Update

Had a chance to review my chart since coming to EHCD and observed the following:

1.   My WBC count at the time of admission to hospital the first time was 3.5 vs. a normal of 4-6 and it now hovers around 1 - I am convinced that my trip to Rochester and the ATG treatments actually caused the WBC count to drop!

2.   My hemoglobin at that time was 7.3 vs. a normal of 15 or better. It now hangs around 9 - 11 depending on how long since my last blood transfusion.

3.   Hematocrits were 19.8 vs. a normal of 30. They now range between 24 and 33.

4.   Platelets were 3,000 vs. a normal of 150,000 - 400,000 (I guess I should have been dead?) The best I have seen since the beginning is 35,000.

The testing here so far has revealed the following that I am about to research more fully:

Elements in my system that are low relative to the general population and/or safe levels:

- Threonine
- Methlhistidine
- Cysteine
- Ammonia
- Methionine
- Amino Acids
- Tyrosine
- Zinc
- Magnesium

Elements that are high relative to the general population and/or safe levels:

- Mercury (probably from dental amalgams),
- Glutamine
- Glycine
- Serine
- Arginine
- Urea

My chart noted something about a glucose-insulin interaction that I need to discuss with Dr. Rea.

I will be meeting with a nutritionist on Monday to discuss what to do now that I know what foods are problematic: Milk, beef, corn, chicken, chocolate, peanuts, shrimp, lobster, cheese, yeasts, eggs, potatoes, oranges, soy, - Is there anything left you ask?

Foods that are okay for me so far: Cabbage (Oh goodie), cane sugar (that's a shock but can't have it due to insulin level), honey, lamb (Yeah!), onions (thank god), pork, strawberries, wheat, ginger, carob, crab, haddock (Doug's Fish Fry here I come), and red peppers. I have a long list of other foods that I will be testing for, but unfortunately most of them are vegetables and I already eat enough of them!

Dinner on Wednesday was butternut squash and cabbage - How wonderful!

The Waiting Game

The amount of time I spend waiting for antigen testing has caused me to think about how much time I have spent waiting since being diagnosed. I have spent more time waiting than ever before in my life.

1. It started with going to Dr. Kirshner office and waiting to be called for my blood draw, then waiting for results and to see Doctor or Kathy. Then waiting to get set up for transfusion. Then waiting in the admitting room to be checked in. Then waiting for whoever is to give me transfusion, then waiting for paperwork, then waiting for meds, then waiting for platelets or blood to show up, then watching the dripping of the IV.

2.	More waiting at BMT unit and hospital. Waiting to see docs, waiting for meds, being awakened at all hours for blood checks. Waiting to go home.

3.	Go to EHCD and watch the clock while I exercise and sauna. Go for testing and wait minutes between tests ("Needles" sticks me about 15-20 times a day and I sit and wait in between sticks with no diversions - no TV, radio, books, computers, etc. and the conversation gets old - BORING!)

4.	Wait for food to cook - Everything has to be cooked from scratch.

I have always been task oriented so this waiting has been a major adjustment but I am surprisingly getting used to it. Not sure how will I adjust back to a more normal life style but would sure like to get the chance!

September 30, 2001 - There is definite hope!

After a bit of a tough day yesterday (felt pretty drained all day but still managed to cook, do laundry and did my full set of PT in the AM), I am feeling great again today. Friday and today I feel almost like my old self. Have a decent amount of energy, my mind is clearer than it has been in a long time and I am hopeful!

Heard very good report on another fund raising event (Poker Run at the riding stables) where we raised a down payment for my sauna (will need to continue this treatment when I go home).

Sue is going to try to sell the house as it would cost too much to retrofit carpeting and it is too much for her to keep up if I am unable to mow lawn (grass reaction) and maintain the pool (loads of harsh chemicals). Very disappointing to think of selling after only living there one summer but what will be, will be.

I have been doing lots of research the last couple of days and my head is clearer than it has been in a long time. Now have gone a full month without needing a blood transfusion. I will have a CBC on Monday with results on Tuesday. Read as part of my research that high altitudes can cause high hematocrits - since mine are low and that is what zaps my energy, should I move to a higher altitude?

Speaking of moving, I am giving serious consideration to relocating to an apartment in a warmer climate. I am very concerned about going back to cold country with all the illnesses that float around in the wintertime in CNY. Maybe we'll have to maintain two smaller homesteads if we can sell the place on Lawsher Drive (we hardly knew ye). The research page and the forum contain all my latest speculation and research.

Lunch today is lettuce and artichoke hearts.

October 3, 2001

I felt pretty weak and tired today - Napped most of the afternoon but beginning to feel a bit stronger again. It has now been over 30 days since blood but did get platelets on Tuesday (counts were P=10, Hemo=8.3, Hematocrits=24, WBC=2.4, RBC=2.4). Have been doing lots of research and discovered a similar disease (actually a Dr. Rea patient has it) called ITP. Have also been dissecting Dr. Young article and discovered in both places the mention of bacteria and viruses as potential causes of AA. I had shingles and have been testing positive to bacteria. Will talk to Dr. Rea about it. Other patients are going through ALF and IV therapy that I also need to ask about it. Settling into a routine of grocery shopping at the organic food store (I do drop by Tom Thumb occasionally for a trip down memory lane), preparing food from scratch and doing dishes like in the old days. I try to catch the 5:30 news but am having a hard time adjusting to that part of the time change. I then spend several hours per day researching and keeping up with the maintenance of the web site. Still nobody else is getting into the research. Everyone seems content to accept whatever the Docs tell him or her and want to keep track of who is dying next. The AA/MDS list is pathetic. Many of the original members have dropped off.

October 7, 2001 – Prepare for checkpoint meeting with Dr. Rea (It's been 7 weeks)

Good News

I feel better than I have in a year

It's been over a month since my last blood transfusion

I can breathe, smell and exercise 30 minutes per day
I am ridding my body of chemical toxins
I am no longer taking all the toxic meds

Bad News

I still need platelets every 7-10 days

I can't make it up a 6-step flight of stairs -Lack of Energy
Still no clear link from immune system to cell growth (CD34 Glycoprotein?)

My immune system is still destroying my blood cells
I am taking more vitamins and supplements than I was meds

Dr. Rea - October 8

Checkpoint Appointment - How are we doing?

No Blood Transfusion since September 2 and then suddenly needed three in one week! Yes, my mind is clearing, I am able to concentrate and my energy level seems to be improving, but still experience fatigue when going up a small flight of stairs. My counts are still not really going anywhere.

I express all this to Dr. Rea and am told that patience is paramount when trying to rebalance the immune system. He admits (for the first time) that he really does not know what will cause my platelets to grow or what will get my red blood cell count in order. His entire focus is on trying to rebalance my immune systems and hopes that this will eventually allow my body to restore the proper blood levels.

I am beginning to realize that this illness is truly my problem and nobody with the possible exception of Sue is going to be really able to do anything. We are going to have to beat this on our own. Dr. Rea may help, but in the end it is going to be up to us!

October 8, 2001 Update

The session with Dr. Rea and Trep went very well. They answered all my questions (see above link) and I may be able to go home if my environment there is safe. (We're working on it) They agree with my statement below and were positively encouraged by my research and approach. For what it's worth, if anyone ever gets to the point of going to the EHCD you really do have to take charge of your own situation. If you are lucky, you get 15 minutes of Dr. Rea once or twice a week and the more research you do on your own (including really reading the reports they give you copies), the better off you will be. He looks at your chart for about 5 minutes a week and it is really up to you to do your homework. I devoured my chart, my independent research and prepared the document mentioned above.

I think everyone is very different and therefore must do the same. Sometimes it is hard to concentrate, but you have to take advantage of the times that you can think and document everything you are trying to do - as

Dr. Rea says, "It's your life - make the time and do the work - what could be more important?" If you are willing to put in the effort, he will help. Otherwise you may as well save your money and stay home. There is "coddling" at the EHCD.

Pretty sure that I am onto something - CD34 presence is significantly reduced in patients with AA. CD34 is somehow linked to Threonine, Cystine and some other amino acid (I'm too tired to look it up). I am low in all of the aforementioned amino acids so will take supplements. Let's see what happens. There is a part of me that believes it couldn't be that simple or one of the brilliant researchers at NIH would have tried it--- but what the heck - I have nothing to lose. My alternative is to continue to get transplants or do a BMT. I am definitely going to exhaust every environmental/natural approach I can find.

October 10, 2001 – Major Set Back

Just when I thought I was making some progress the roof fell in again. I was all psyched up thinking the environment clinical depuration therapy stuff was working and then my counts went lower than they have ever been. Crits dropped to 16 and Hemoglobin to 6.7. That is lower than when I had my original episode and even after 4 units of packed red blood cells they just barely crept into the safe range again. I had a temperature of 102, cold sweats and chills and could barely walk by the time I arrived at St. Paul's Hospital in Dallas

Very disappointing. Will continue with the EHCD regimen but this was a blow to my confidence. Have been in the hospital for the past two days getting blood, platelets and Desferol with a roommate that had the TV on all day with visitors talking over the top of the TV -What a joy! Up and down we go, round and round we go. Going on 10 months of this fun.

October 12, 2001 - Feeling Really Good Again

In this never ending up and down battle I felt really good and energized today. Like I should feel after getting 4 units of blood and 1 unit of platelets but the counts not responding very well definitely has me puzzled. I took two doses of Calmax from James today, did 30 minutes solid on the treadmill, 30 minutes of sauna and had IV therapy of all essential vitamins, minerals and amino acids plus extra on Vitamin C and a few others. I was unable to buy Threonine locally so ordered it online for delivery to Syracuse (hope I'm back there soon). Will buy Cystine and arginine tomorrow. My appointment with Dr. Rea originally scheduled for Wednesday is now tomorrow at 9:45 and we decide if I should go home or not considering the crash episode of Tuesday/Wednesday. I'm not sure what to do - Sick of being here but if another few days would help I will likely stick it out. Need to try to meet with Dr. Griffis (Immunologist/Microbiologist) to discuss my CD34 Threonine theory.

October 18 Update - "The Truth - Always the Truth"

I just spent another night in the hospital - My best guess is that I have spent well over two months now in a hospital bed and another two months in a crummy cotton covered piece of plywood all in hopes of finding some way of beating Aplastic Anemia. Today, I would have to say that AA is winning. My counts are actually worse than they were when I started and that is after SIX units of blood and FOUR units of platelets. This is not progress!!

After a little over a week since getting both blood and platelets by platelets were at 5000 (the lowest they have ever been!) and a week ago, my other counts were at their lowest ever. I am angry, discouraged, disappointed but still determined to beat this damn thing. What I am realizing more than ever is that nobody is going to do it for me. My only hope rests in working with my wife on trying to make something in the whole world of natural healing work while continuing to research and try to find my own cure.

In summary, I am pretty disappointed at the moment. I have spent nearly $20,000 and my counts are no better than when the day I arrived at the Environmental Health Center of Dallas. I may be impatient, but it would seem to me that after over two months of eating a restrictive diet, getting poked in the arm an average of 15-20 times a day, "depurating" (exercise, sauna, massage), taking God knows how many tests, IV Therapy, Oxygen Therapy and virtually everything they offered, my counts would have improved. THEY DID NOT!

Now, if my objective had been to detoxify and "balance my immune system", then I would have to say that it probably worked and may even recommend the place to others, but at least for now, I would have a very hard time recommending it to anyone who has a serious disease like AA. Most of the people here have allergies or have somehow been exposed to toxins and or chemicals, and more than a few are just whacko. I needed to get out of here before I became one of them!

Earlier on we did some heavy speculation as to the cause of my illness. Sue's original theory about me popping fertilizer laden golf balls is still her most prominent theory. I consider others like the mercury that was released into my system during extensive dental work in the past several months prior to being diagnosed. I have also read that Aplastic Anemia and Autoimmune disease can be caused by excessive use of antibiotics.

I was prescribed many different antibiotics over the years in an effort to combat my almost annual bout with sore throats. I also received heavy doses of penicillin and other drugs for my childhood meningitis. Or maybe, the shingle episode about ten years ago may have triggered my immune system to begin overreacting?

Others have speculated that benzene is a likely cause or they attribute blame to the toxins and chemicals that are found everywhere in our modern society. Molds and pollens are believed to trigger allergic reactions and the formaldehyde that is commonly found in building materials (and therefore malls) is a definite suspect. I have also been almost constantly exposed to natural gas. Radon is prevalent in the area where we live and I have certainly been overexposed to paints and varnishes in all the building activities over the years. Some recent suspects include a pellet stove in our new house and the incredible stress associated with starting a new business. Any or all of these could be causes or contributing factors.

It is now apparent however, that all the speculation in the world is not going to change the indisputable fact that I am sick and am not going to get well until I can get my immune system in balance. The only thing that matters now is trying to figure out some way to get my counts back to normal and before I can even think about doing that I have to get my strength back and that will not happen until my immune system gets back on balance.

After nearly three months in Texas, we have returned full circle to the challenges of deciding what foods to eat or not, what to eliminate from my environment and what changes to make in my lifestyle. I reluctantly decide to remove myself from the business and Melissa takes full control.

The regimen at the EHCD was designed to get my immune system back in balance through the use of antigen shots, a rotational diet and detoxification program that included a physical therapy program and a daily sauna.

I later developed my own strategy based on this regimen and believe that it has been instrumental in returning me to a normal lifestyle.

My strategy includes a good exercise program (at least 30 minutes a day using various stretching, walking and light weights), lots of fresh air and sunshine. I eat mostly "grains, greens and bean" which means I eat a lot of lettuce, rice and beans of various sorts. I take a multivitamin daily. I went through a period where I was taking more vitamins and supplements than I had been taking medications but have now tapered off everything except the multiple and the supplements necessary to replace nutrients depleted during the sauna.

I have learned to listen to my body and am now able to eat the foods necessary to keep it functioning properly. I am still heavily "grains, greens and beans" based and eat a banana every day to keep my potassium level where it belongs. I also occasionally will eat small quantities of select meat, fish or eggs for protein. I drink plenty of fresh spring water and eat lots of carrots and fruit. More detailed information on my approach is available in the chapter on Holistic Medicine.

Now, forever implanted in the memory brain cells associated with the assassination, there is new entry for a rejuvenating but costly trip to Dallas and the EHCD.

Another version of the EHCD experience is available at http://www.ehcd.com/websteen/dallas_trip.htm. Address for the EHCD is 8345 Walnut Hill Lande, Suite 220, Dallas, TX 75231 and phone number is 214-368-4132.

Chapter 17

Laying on Of Hands

The Divine Transfusion

Probably one of the reasons I took to nicknaming myself is that I didn't particularly like the handles being bestowed upon me by childhood "friends." "Tiger" was acceptable because it spoke to my aggressive nature on the athletic field and "Big Fella" fit my 6'3", 150-pound gangly frame. I did not much care for "Bones" as the alternate description of that same frame and "90 Pound Weakling" was the least favorite of my derisive handles.

"Bones" was the favorite moniker chosen by my boyhood tormentor and town bully, Lowell Schluter (funny how I remember those names with hatred after over thirty years). One late August day on the fairway of the 8th hole of Appleton's municipal golf course, Lowell had me in a stranglehold and was pummeling me with his fists when my best buddy, Rich Melin came out of nowhere and within minutes had the kid screaming in pain.

"Toad" as Rich was unfortunately labeled and will be remembered until there are no members of the Appleton High School Class of '66 still alive, had the kid tied up in a half nelson and made this kid promise to leave me alone or he would break his arm. From that day forward, Mr. Town bully was very careful not to even give me a dirty look, let alone use the dreaded nickname for fear of losing his arm.

Rich was the equipment manager for both football and basketball and the self-appointed lead booster especially when we were on the road. I still remember him urging me on in his own special style - "Come on Tiger, you can do it."

As with many childhood friendships, Rich and I drifted apart over the years. He was a groomsman in our wedding and we even managed to get the families together a few times but when Rich and his wife, Sally moved to Oklahoma, we even lost track of a proper address. Rich put himself through medical school at the incredible age of 42 and was practicing his own special brand of healing somewhere on an Indian Reservation we thought.

When Sue learned that we would be in Texas at the EHCD, she tracked down our old friends, and just like on the golf course so many years earlier, Rich came charging to the rescue like David ready to slay Goliath. He had always been much more religious than I was. He and Sally sometimes made me a bit uncomfortable with their proclamations of how Jesus was at the center of their lives.

Yes, I was a Christian, but when Rich and I sang in the youth choir together, I kept my conservative Midwestern Lutheran witnessing to a minimum. Garrison Keillor could have easily based his Prairie Home Companion series on the Lutheran churches of my youth.

Without a moment's hesitation, Rich and Sally made arrangements to meet in a small town between Dallas and Oklahoma City. Since it was a Sunday, they wondered if we would want to join them for a church service.

Unknown to me at the time, Sue and Sally had carefully orchestrated this little charade and before I knew it, I was encircled by Rich and a small group of the "Church Elders" who were mumbling in strange tongues seeking God's blessing for this "child of God."

It was a bit like a scene from Robert Duvall's "Apostle", but I truly felt the power of God enter my body as Rich prayed for a Divine Transfusion." No, I did not become a "Born Again Christian," but the overwhelming experience caused me to strengthen my belief in the Almighty and to renew my commitment to serve Him with the remainder of my life here on earth, however long that may be.

It may have taken a bit longer than I expected, but that "Divine Transfusion" did work and I credit Rich, Sally and my best friend in the whole world for helping me get my spiritual house in order. As she had so often done in the past, Sue was working her own brand of miracle.

As a devout Catholic when we met, Sue made me promise that we would raise our children in a Christian manner. I readily agreed, but as time went on, I began to drift further and further from the Church. In an effort to bring us closer together and strengthen our relationship with God, she gave up her childhood faith to become a Lutheran.

I did not fully comprehend it at the time, but this was an incredible sacrifice on her part and her faith has helped us weather many a storm. Catholics honestly believe that theirs is the "one true faith" and once you leave the Catholic Church you will be prohibited from entering heaven. For Sue to go against this teaching was incomprehensible to many, but she did it knowing in her heart that it was the best thing for the family.

Our spiritual well-being was critical then and is even more so today as we deal with the stresses surrounding my illness.

Irish Blessing

May the road rise up to meet you.
May the wind be always at your back
The sunshine warm upon your face,
The rain fall soft upon your fields,
And until we meet again
May God hold you in the hollow of His hand.

* * * * *

Shortly after our visit with Rich and Sally, Sue returned to her work as a school nurse. Her boss had been very understanding throughout our ordeal, but it was time for Sue to try to return to something resembling a normal life. Before she left, she stocked the cupboards and left me specific menus. She is certainly the best caretaker in the world!

I managed okay and my life settled into boring routine. I awoke at 7:00am, walked to the Center, checked in and did my exercise and sauna. By 9:00 I was in the needle room enduring an average of 10 test shots per day. I walked back to the condo for lunch and returned for more testing. Some days I would do the sauna regimen in the afternoon also.

Returning to the condo around 5:00, I would fix my dinner watch a few hours of TV and retire for the night. Every day was pretty much the same routine broken only by an occasional visit to the Whole Food Market to select my predetermined menus.

Since my environment had been limited to about a one square mile area, I decided to venture out a little. One day, I visited the local Guitar Center and implemented a time-honored tradition -I pretended to be interested in purchasing a new "axe" and spent several nearly uninterrupted hours entertaining myself. I have actually purchased a new guitar once in a while, but most often use this little routine when I have been away from my own guitars for an extended time.

On the weekend I ventured into downtown, had my first meal out in over a month and visited the famous grassy knoll and library warehouse that has made Dallas a city with a past. It is interesting how we remember where we were and what we doing on certain days in our lives. I vividly recall the day President Kennedy was shot. I was in my high school Biology class and spent the next several days glued to the TV witnessing the murder of Lee Harvey Oswald and the funeral.

Chapter 18

All Things Considered

I Would Rather Die at Home

For the third or fourth time in less than a year, I had faced the very real possibility of my own death. I was not particularly frightened by any of the experiences and was determined to win my battle with AA one way or another.

It would be safe to say that my battle was not going well. By now, I had tried ATG and ALG. I had been given the interleukin-2 and other "growth hormone shots," had ingested the dreadful Cyclosporine for almost a year.

I had seen first-hand what a Bone Marrow Transplant could do to someone when we met other patients in St Louis and I read the real statistics online. I had tried the alternative treatment protocol espoused by Drs. Rogers and Rea.

As I said before, what started as an almost interesting encounter had turned into a battle for my life and we were desperate enough to try almost any thing

I did not fully comprehend the serious nature of my illness until I was officially diagnosed as "non-responsive" to the two rounds or therapeutic ATG/ALG treatments. I was fighting and losing in the battle to regain control of my everyday life. I became weaker every day and was caught in a devastating catch-22.

My blood could not support exercise and the more days that went by without exercise the weaker I became. Then faced with the most important decision of my life. Should I go for a transplant or not? If so, where should I have it? And probably most important, when or how long do I wait? When I finally pressed the

BMT center at Strong Memorial for their success rate with Aplastic Anemia patients I learned they were 0 for 5!!

We also met a woman of a former AA Strong patient while in St. Louis whose son died at the center. As much as we loved the people and had been impressed by the care, we were beginning to lose faith in the possibility of a positive outcome of a Bone Marrow Transplant. I also had done some research online and discovered that Strong was not alone in their number of failures, and as the old saying goes, doctors bury their mistakes.

Stem cell research has a potentially direct impact on AA/MDS/PNH specifically because when you have a BMT, you are really only receiving stem cells (the other cells die off and you are left with the stem cells) in all types of BMT - BMT, PBSC, Cord Blood Stem Cell.

Warning - This is the section of "Life According to Bubba" in which I will discuss my political views and air my feelings regarding how pharmaceutical companies are controlling modern medicine. - If you or your small children are offended by religious or political debate, please proceed with caution!

From P, 5, of "What Doctors Don't Tell You" by Lynne McTaggart ISBN 0-380-79607-4

"One glance at the statistics shows that, except in the case of getting run over or needing an emergency cesarean, orthodox Western medicine not only won't cure you but may leave you worse off than you were before. In fact, these days, scientific medicine itself is responsible for a good percentage of disease. If you're in a hospital, there's a one in six chance that you landed there because of some modern medical treatment gone wrong.4 Once you get there, your chances are one in six of dying in the hospital or suffering some injury while you're there. Since a doctor or hospital's error causes half this risk, you've got an 8 percent chance of being killed or injured by the staff5.

Each footnote cited by Ms. McTaggart sites a reputable source and although her conclusions may be a bit overstated, anyone entering a hospital or in the care of a doctor needs to exercise due diligence. In essence, it is about balancing risk vs. reward.

For the record, I am not against doctors. I am convinced that most doctors mean well and I know for a fact that at least one of them saved my life in a critical care situation. I am however, convinced that ATG and Cyclosporine did me more harm than good. I also believe that prescription medicine has become far too prevalent and alternative treatments should be considered.

In addition to my readings on the history of civilization, I did some research into the history of modern medicine. Although there are many lifesaving advances that we should be grateful for, there are also some remedies and strategies that should be questioned.

My obvious personal question is whether or not the current treatment protocol for Aplastic Anemia is in fact the appropriate one.

1.   BMT appears to be high risk - At best, the survival rate appears to be less than 40% in adults over 50.

2.   On the other side, the more transplants you have, the more there is a chance of building up antibodies that will reject future transplant and/or transfusions.

3.   Most reading suggests that I only do a BMT if nothing else works. Other reading suggests that if you are going to do a BMT, you do it as early as possible with the least number of transfusions.

I had applied for long-term medical disability with Social Security* and was approved in almost record time. This was both a blessing and a curse. The SS agent told me that I had been "fast-tracked" and I had to wonder why. Why would the SSA approve me so quickly? What did they know that I did not? Was I going to die in less than two years?

*Social Security Administration 1-800-772-1213

I considered what would be best for my wife and family regarding the house we live in, the prospect that I may never work full time again and made my spiritual peace. I had countless hours to contemplate, read, journalize and discover my attitudes and philosophies. I had always been too busy "doing" to spend time thinking and researching.

I realized that this was a chance to "flesh out" my personal philosophy of life and seek the knowledge and understanding that had heretofore eluded me. I started with real interesting conversations with the people closest to me - my wife, my daughters, my best friend, Jack and others. I learned from Jack that he did believe in God, but was vehemently opposed to organized religion.

I began reading serious non-fiction starting with the History of Knowledge, The Ascent of Man, 100 Most Influential People in the World and numerous medically oriented books including "How We Die", "Commotion in the Blood", "The Rebellious Body" to name a few. On Sue's recommendation, and conclusions formed in my readings, I began to research the cause of my illness and finally agreed with her that it could be "Multiple Chemical Sensitivities" or "MCS."

I had politely (sometimes not so politely) observed her incredible research into the true causes for many modern illnesses. She had by now read all of Dr. Sherry Rogers's books and many others that espouse how our toxic chemically laden environment is the root cause for virtually every modern illness. I also encountered several interesting websites including ones by Dr. Stoll and Dr. Weill who set forward the same theories. Early on, these beliefs seemed pretty far-fetched, but since nothing else seemed to be working for me, I was now ready to at least try an "alternative approach."

I taught myself to become a better researcher and documented everything on the web site or on one of my computers (I am a practicing "techno-freak" with a handheld, laptop and several desktop computers.)

In addition to the "hard facts", I also tried to pay more attention to the subtleties around me. I developed friendships with caretakers and promised myself to be more aware of the needs of others, especially fellow patients, most of who had previously suffered in silence. Through the web site and the message forums, I continue to challenge people to become more involved.

Our own local efforts began with a golf tournament, press releases and virtually anything we could do to bring awareness to my personal plight and the plight of others diagnosed with AA and MDS. I questioned my own motives at times and wrestled with putting my business and marketing knowledge into what was essentially a personal problem. I vividly remember Sue saying, "you're a salesman for God's sake - sell it!"

In the end, I took her advice, guidance from the Aplastic Anemia International Foundation and my friend Jack. I resolved that this was not a time to be shy. When you are in a battle for your life, you need to use every weapon at your disposal! The number of special people who came to my aid was incredible. I have always been essentially a non-feeling and aloof personality.

I considered myself to be a leader and motivator but lacked the true caring nature of a true leader. Hopefully this experience will teach me a valuable lesson about the needs of others. Beginning with my wife, Sue who has been by my side for over thirty years through the good times and the bad. She endured countless hours of my verbal abuse and frustration, cared for my physical, mental and emotional needs and helped me understand what was happening.

She re-launched her own personal research into the immune system, chemical sensitivity and environmental illness rekindling the painful experience associated with Michelle and her long battles.

Through it all, she was supportive, consoling and loving beyond belief. My daughters also rose to the occasion and helped me realize what a wonderful job Sue had done in raising them. Sure, I was around, but they received their nurturing and guidance from their mother. When the chips were down, it was her guidance that manifested itself in their caring and assistance to me.

Upon finally realizing that the medical community was probably not going to provide a durable cure for my Aplastic Anemia, I resolved to treat myself. Sue actually led the charge in the same manner she had tackled Michelle's illness so many years ago. She dug out her old books on Environmental Illness, arranged to see Dr. Sherry Rogers, and helped me to see the light. My absolute best chance at beating this awful disease is to go after the root cause.

Stop just throwing lethal drugs at it and find out what can be done to rebuild my immune system so that it works properly. I now firmly believe that my situation is the result of chemical overload. I am not yet sure what should be done, but will begin by detoxifying my body and going on a macrobiotic diet.

Chapter 19

A Temperature of 106.4!

Did Anybody See that Truck?

The Centers for Disease Control and Prevention estimates that 2 million people annually acquire infections while hospitalized and 90,000 people die from those infections. More than 70 percent of hospital-acquired infections have become resistant to at least one of the drugs commonly used to treat them, largely due to the over prescribing of antibiotics by physicians.

Staph, the leading cause of hospital infections, is now resistant to 95 percent of first-choice antibiotics and 30 percent of second-choice antibiotics. Poor staff hygiene is considered the leading source for infections acquired during hospitalizations. But efforts to get medical workers to improve safety through things as simple as better and more frequent hand washing have met with little success.

April 21, 2002 - - Record Temperature of 106.4

Shortly after my return from the strange trip to Rochester, I began to feel something was not right again. My temp went up a little on Tuesday night and a truck parked in my driveway. Wednesday morning it ran me over.

I made it to Nurse Klinger long enough to confirm that my temperature was 102 degrees and rising. I had to leave their office by ambulance and arrived at good ol' CGH at 2:00 Wednesday PM. It took forever to get me checked in (my pal Judy had obviously departed for the day as she usually streamlines the process before I even arrive).

I finally made it to a bed about 3:00 only to be greeted by a nurse who had that look I had learned to fear. She could care less about me and just wanted to get out of there for the day. A hospital can be a frightening place when you are alone (Sue was still at work and did not realize how serious this had become).

It was shift change time and from past experience I knew that was the absolute worst time to arrive on a floor. A word of advice - Never be seriously ill at 3:00 P.M, 11:00 P.M. or 7:00 AM.

Miss "I just want to get out of here" took my temperature in each ear and it registered 105 both times. She mumbled that this couldn't be right and then took it orally (right after I drank some ice water) and it registered 103. "There that's better, I'll chart 103, "says she with a triumphant smile.

She also mentioned I may have to use the cooling blanket machine and I in my delirious state, said "Oh, no, not that." That was enough for her to chart that I had refused the cooling blanket. Secure in her diagnoses and leaving me close to death, she filled out her chart and went home.

The cooling blanket is a refrigerator for humans. You lie on a plastic sheet filled with cold water and the machine keeps it refrigerated. You pretty much feel like you are lying on an ice rink without your clothes for protection; hence my "refusal" because I had endured this once before. Would anyone in their right mind "refuse" the cooling blanket if it would keep them alive?

By this time, I was having tremors and pretty much delirious. At 4:00, my evening nurse showed up and observed that golly my temp was really 106.2! (Sue told me later that I should have had a seizure and died at that level.)

Nurse number two brought in the cooling blanket but couldn't get it to work. By that time my pulse was 99 and my blood pressure was 89 over 47. . Finally my hero Kristine arrived took charge and said, "Whoa, we have to get this thing under control. My temp topped out at 106.4 (I believe that to be a new world's record for old farts who live to tell about it).

She got the cooling blanket working added some ice packs and finally got things under control. I could have easily been a victim of patient neglect but was so out of it during the process I really didn't even know what was happening.

The next day, they pulled my infected line and I began to feel like I might live. I have really had enough of these shakeups! Thank God Sue was by my side and insisted people do their jobs or I probably would have bought the farm, ranch and entire state of Texas. No more trucks please!

I pretty much lost an entire couple of days and returned to my normal AA status (light headed, lousy counts and great attitude) (Yuk!) My PICC line had staph infection and had to be pulled so I will now have my fifth central line installed (I think - I kind of lose track of these things).

This was my fourth near death experience and when I was discharged this time, I vowed it would not happen again. I made the final decision to get on an alternative treatment program.

In subsequent days I leaned that I had septicemia* (blood infection). The doctor who removed my PICC line said that she could actually see the virus sticking to the end of my PICC line.

The infectious control doctor for the hospital got involved very quickly and Sue said it was because they didn't want a lawsuit. She was quite sure that my infection was the result of poor technique and suspected a nurse she had noticed with long fingernails. Germs love to hide under the fingernails.

*Septicemia is the presence of bacteria in the blood (bacteremia) and is often associated with severe disease.

Septicemia is a serious, rapidly progressive, life-threatening infection that can arise from infections throughout the body, including infections in the lungs, abdomen, and urinary tract. Septicemia can rapidly lead to septic shock and death.

The chart below shows what my counts were three days after receiving a transfusion:

	Mine	Normal Range
White Blood Cells	1.3K	4.8 – 10.8
Red Blood Cells	2.79	4.7 – 6.1
Hemoglobin	10	14-18
Platelets	15K	150-400K

My potassium and several other chemistry levels were extremely low so I needed a few supplements before I could be discharged.

Earlier in my diagnosis I checked a book out of the library called "How We Die" by Dr. Sherwin Nuland. He explains that death is attributed to many and varied causes, but the ultimate culprit in nearly all cases is heart failure or technically "cardiac ischemia." Ischemia is described as a low oxygen state due to obstruction of the arterial blood supply or inadequate blood flow leading to hypoxia in the tissue.

"The afflicted patient becomes increasingly short of breath with even minimal exertion, since neither the heart nor the lungs can respond to the increase in the work demanded of them. Some sufferers have difficult lying down for more than a short period of time because they need the upright position and gravity to drain excess fluid from their lungs.

I have known many patients for who sleep became impossible unless their head and shoulders were elevated on several pillows

And even then they were subject to paroxysms of frightening breathlessness during the night.

Patients in heart failure suffer also from chronic fatigue and listlessness, owing to a complication of the added effort of simply breathing and the poor tissue nutrition caused by low cardiac output. "

In essence, my red blood cells are incapable of carrying the necessary oxygen to muscles, brain and other organs.

"As the blood count and flow continues to diminish, the patient will literally starve and ultimately destroy the vital organs of the liver, kidneys and heart. The patient will became jaundice, suffer uremia and die."

I had nearly experienced this complete failure five times and finally decided to take full charge of my own destiny. I had somewhat blindly trusted my life to others and it was not working. I am still convinced that most medical professionals don't mean to do harm but because of understaffing and a lack of knowledge do ultimately become responsible for a large portion of the deaths in hospitals every year.

From P, 5, of "What Doctors Don't Tell You" by Lynne McTaggart

"One glance at the statistics shows that, except in the case of getting run over or needing an emergency cesarean, orthodox Western medicine not only won't cure you but may leave you worse off than you were before. In fact, these days, scientific medicine itself is responsible for a good percentage of disease. If you're in a hospital, there's a one in six chance that you laded there because of some modern medical treatment gone wrong. Once you get there, your chances are one in six of dying in the hospital or suffering some injury while you're there.

Since a doctor or hospital's error causes half this risk, you're got an 8 percent chance of being killed or injured by the staff. If we extrapolate the results of a 1984 study, over one million Americans are being injured in the hospital every year, and 180,000 die as a result. To put the magnitude of the problem in perspective, if you live in the United States, where about 40,000 people are shot dad every year, you are nevertheless three times more likely to be killed by a doctor than by a gun. This appalling track record has nothing to do with incompetence or lack of dedication. Most doctors are extremely well intended, and probably a majority is competent in what they've been taught.

The problem is not the carpenter, but his tools. The fact is that medicine is not a science, or even an art. Many of your doctor's arsenal of treatments don't work - indeed have never been proven to work, let alone to be safe. It is a false science, built upon conjuring tricks, supposition, and blind preconception, where so-called scientific method is a vast amount of stumbling in the dark."

The second leading cause of the ultimate death is pneumonia because the blood can't keep circulating properly and fluid fills the lungs literally suffocating the patient to death on their own fluids. The technical term is "acute pulmonary edema" - "the presence of abnormally large amounts of fluid in the intercellular tissue spaces of the lungs usually followed by an accumulation of excessive fluid in the subcutaneous tissues."

During my first hospitalization in Rochester, I experienced this first hand when my lungs began to fill with fluid and my ankles swelled to twice their normal size. According to Dr. Nuland, this swelling is caused by pressure from the vena cava to veins. The blood is incapable of returning the waste products accumulated in the blood back to the heart for cleansing so they build up in other areas of the body.

My fluid buildup was also the result of "overdosing" on IV fluids. My "know it all" resident at the time kept pumping me full of fluids even when Sue told her that my ankles were swelling. Sue insisted on another doctor being called and when the pulmonary specialist showed up the very first thing she did was cut the IV fluids. I was better in a matter of a few hours!

I vividly remember her using the term "pulmonary edema" and my cause of death for this episode would have been listed as "acute pulmonary edema" when in fact it was due to a resident, or whatever she was, being too arrogant to do the right thing even after being told by an RN with over thirty years of experience that something was not right.

I had by now arrived at some key conclusions:

1.	Trusting the caretakers could cost me my life!
2.	I would do everything I could to keep my heart as strong as possible
3.	I would exercise my upper body and keep my lungs clear
4.	I would find a better way of combating my illness than being in hospitals
5.	Hospitals are where people go to die!

In the summary to his book, Dr. Nuland offers this clinical description of the death of one of his first patients:

"The man's coronary arteries were unable to bring sufficient blood to nourish the muscles of his heart, the heartbeat became ineffective, the brain went too long without oxygen, and the man died. This was a simple culmination of a straight forward series of biological events."

Unfortunately, my aplastic anemia is accelerating this natural biological progression because of my inability to supply the much-needed oxygen to all the parts of my body. My brain is not functioning properly; my heart is pounding from overwork and my legs cramp up due to poor circulation. I have persistent "neuropathy" in my feet. Due to the lack of oxygen, the nerves in my feet are literally starved and I have no sense of feel. My feet feel like they are already dead. I need to find a way to stop this progression and get my life back.

To be clear, I abused my body for well over thirty years. No doctor or hospital was responsible for my illness. Doctors saved my life and the hospital had what was necessary to make that happen. But it is now up to me to make myself better. I must take better care of myself and develop a program to help my body heal itself.

I had committed myself to an exercise program from the beginning but I was now determined to extend the exercise even though it meant taxing my heart a bit. My only real concern here was that I would tax it so much that it would collapse. I talked to Nurse Klinger and she said to be careful, not run or lift heavy weights but otherwise the concept was a good one.

Chapter 20

Conventional Medicine

Stories from the Frontlines

"I used to live my life with the windows rolled up and the radio blaring, tuning out life as I drove along. But I was lucky enough to get that little nudge from God that makes me roll down the windows and look at the incredible beauty that life is. Getting AA did that for me."

Mindy Pember - A Member of Aplastic Central Web Forum

Mindy and I ultimately disagreed on a course of treatment but her attitude and help was instrumental in my decision to combat the illness with everything I had. She came along at a time when I was beginning to lose hope and helped me to see that there were ways to beat this ugly thing. Mindy was (and is) as she says, "one of the lucky ones" who is now a card carrying, back packing survivor of Aplastic Anemia. Through my web site, I have had the pleasure of meeting people from all over the world.

Aplastic Anemia (or any life altering illness) is certainly not for the weak in spirit. It is a devastating, debilitating and frightening illness that has killed far too many people. These illnesses will test you to your very core. You will be tested physically, emotionally and spiritually in ways you never imagined.

I am particularly frustrated by the lack of progress in fighting these illness and for somewhat obvious reasons have now chosen to dedicate a large part of my life to finding a cure for Aplastic Anemia, MDS and the other autoimmune related diseases. I have moved beyond the central issue of beating the illness for my own purposes and now want to prevent these illnesses from taking any more lives.

One of my latest correspondents is from the Faroe Islands:

"Dear Bruce, My name is Jonna. My daughter Mia is 23 years old and has had AA since September. 1998. We live in Faroe Islands, between Iceland and Norway in the Atlantic sea. I am not good to write English, but I will try. Mia was 19 year old when she was diagnosed with severe AA. She have ATG (horse) 3 x, and she have taken Cyclosporine first 2 year - then no medication for 1 year - and so here count beginning to go dawn - so she started again with Cyclosporine, but she had so many side effect and now she started with Mycophenolate Mofetil (MMF) also known as CellCept- and it is much milder - now here count are very fine. She work every day - and live a normal life. Thank you for this AA homepage - is very good for us - in the Faroe Island is Mia the only patient whit AA - so we feel very lonely. There live 45.000 people here - and there are 18 islands. Please - if you have time - write to us :))"

Nearly every story begins with a statement similar to this one from Erica:

"I got diagnosed with severe aplastic anemia in January 2000. It was the first time I ever heard of this disease. It was the first I was really ill and in a hospital for it. So there were loads of new experiences for me. I was treated with ATG, G-CSF, Cyclosporine and lots of all kinds of medications. The ATG seemed to be working and in September I was going to college again, taking things slow. Things went better, my Cyclosporine less and my trust more. Until the beginnings of June my blood cell-counts had dropped and the Cyclosporine went back to 275 mg a day. This was a big disappointment. I just got used with being a student instead of a patient again and now I was back where I started. Now, half July, my counts have stopped dropping; the bone marrow shows nothing funny, other than having aplastic anemia. Today, it was thirteen days ago I had my last transfusion with platelets and my hematologist (Dr. Barge from Leiden Medical Centre) is optimistic. I am in good spirit and I believe I will get better.

In January of 2001, shortly after my diagnosis, I decided to start a website to capture the information I was researching on the Internet. As a side note, I have been using the Internet since the days before there was a Graphical User Interface (GUI). I was one of the first 10,000 users of America Online - I know that because back then you had a user number instead of a user name.

I almost immediately said to myself, self - this is really cool! As another side note, I later attended a seminar where a presenter remarked, "If you were one of the first users of this grand new technology and did not invest in AOL, you're as dumb as a rock." It is a humbling experience to admit to one's supreme ignorance!

So, anyway, I decided to capture my thoughts online and then broadened it into a place where others could do the same if they were inclined to do so. Aplastic Central now receives an average of 500 hits per day from people all over the world. They share their stories, read mine, talk to each other and read the hundreds of pages of assembled information. It is a gratifying experience that has consumed many thousand hours of my time and the time of countless other contributors.

The Aplastic Central members deserve a lot of the credit because without them, this venture would not have continued. In addition to the many messages expressing frustration, loss and fear there were a like number of notes discussing successes, treatments to try, and welcome notes of encouragement.

When things go wrong, as they sometimes will,

When the road you're trudging seems all up hill,
When the funds are low and the debts are high,

And you want to smile, but you have to sigh,
When care is pressing you down a bit,
Rest, if you must - but don't you quit.

Anonymous

As a patient, one of the most important aspects in the treatment strategy you choose is your own personal attitude. It is absolutely critical to surround yourself with positive people and positive thoughts as you deal with the daily stresses or your illness and the disruption it will bring into your life and the lives of the people you love.

As mentioned previously I have a very real respect for the good caretakers. One of my favorites has been nicknamed my Advocate General and she carefully monitors my progress on a weekly basis. Nurse Klinger, as I call her, not only takes my pulse, checks my vitals and charts my progress, but also takes an active interest in how I am coping with my illness. She and many others are on the constant watch for the first signs of an infection, any unusual bleeding or bruising and any emotional changes.

They know from experience that what may seem minor to me could quickly lead to a serious complication. Sue is also ever vigilant insisting that I report any and all aberrations. I have experienced several close calls already with "serum disease" in March and a serious blood infection in late August. I literally "saw the light" while fighting off the serum disease and have been much more cautious since the sepsis infection raised my temperature to 106 degrees.

It is very easy to develop a feeling of hopelessness and began a period of self-pity. It took a while for me to realize it, but the strain on family members and especially those closest to me was even more telling. While we as patients are lying in a comfortable (ok - not always so comfortable) hospital bed, our loved ones are being forced to deal with the emotional and physical strains of life without us.

Life still must go on. Shopping for food, shoveling the snow (or mowing the grass if you are fortunate enough to live somewhere other than Central New York), and all the otherwise normal daily chores still must be done. And on top of these extra burdens, our loved ones are dealing with medical bills, phone calls from well-wishing friends, and constantly putting on a "brave face" for you.

The strain at times is unbelievable and just when there appears to be relief in sight, the patient takes an unexpected turn and it begins all over again in earnest. Just when it appeared that I may be "out of the woods" following a hopeful visit to the BMT center in Rochester, I contracted a blood infection from my central line and was back at Community General in Syracuse again fighting for my life.

The strain was now highly visible on Sue's face and for the first time, I realized that my illness was taking more out of her and Melissa than it was out of me. They were the ones doing battle behind the scenes with the insurance companies, the medical bills, the late night phone calls, the early morning doctor's visits, the twenty-four hour hospital room vigils sleeping in very uncomfortable recliners, and the constant fear that I may not be with them tomorrow.

One of the most important things that everyone who is battling a life altering illness needs is hope and this absolutely includes the support team. Early on I was determined not to let "my" website become a place for people to commiserate and "swap sappy stories." It was going to be a content oriented site focusing on facts and research. (Sue and my omniscient friend Jack sort of smiled at this declaration and it wasn't until much later that it dawned on me that they sensed from the beginning that the site would provide much needed therapy for so many people - including yours truly).

I eventually realized how vitally important it was for the readers to share their fears, successes and failures. The forum has become a sounding board for the hundreds of people who now visit the site on a regular basis.

The website also includes a member's stories area that features over two hundred personal accounts of how patients and loved ones are facing this illness. Even though the contributors are battling their own personal demons, nearly every story is hopeful and upbeat.

There are others that will tear your heart out like the ones from desperate mothers and fathers who have just learned that their infant child has AA or some similar illness. They are distraught, worried and desperate for answers. I help as best I can and offer to pray for them, but what can one say when a child succumbs to an early illness. I received several emails like this one:

"Our hematologist seems to think our daughter may have AA but has not diagnosed her yet. She has a bone marrow test on Friday morning. I have been reading up since he talked to us this morning to try and educate myself. Our doctor mentioned this is a worst-case scenario so I am a little interested as to what that means. He would not go into specifics with us today because he wants to see all the tests. Her hemoglobin was at 2.1 last night so they rushed her to PICU. It all has happened so fast. I am praying often and will continue researching. My daughter is 2 months old so the doctor is very confused as she is very young. I would like to get on a mailing list for news about this disease and also any advice or good questions to ask the doctors would be appreciated. Thanks."

Another from a mother who will never forget the devastation AA caused in her life:

"I have just finished reading your battle with this awful disease and admire your determination to beat it. Bruce, in 1961 my darling son, aged four, died within three months of diagnosis. There was no real treatment way back then. It grieves me to think that, with all the advances in medicine, there is still no guaranteed cure. I write this with a heavy heart - one really never gets over the death of a child. No doubt here, in Australia, research is still going on and patients battling with AA just as you are doing. Keep the fight going - your story will encourage other sufferers I'm sure. God bless you."

Reading these stories somehow has motivated me to work harder at finding a cure or a way to deal with the dreadful consequences of autoimmune disorders. By this time, I had moved from Aplastic Anemia to a more generalized class of illnesses that seem to all have at their root the malfunctioning of the immune system.

I had learned that one of the fundamental problems with Aplastic Anemia is that our bodies' immune system destroys the blood cells before they are allowed to enter the blood stream. (Please see the chapter on research for a thorough discussion on the causes and potential cures for AA-MDS and other Autoimmune Disorders).

Most times, I respond privately to emails, but occasionally will ask to share the story on the Aplastic Central Readers' Forum. Most first time writers are frightened and frustrated with the lack of real information available to people who suffer from Aplastic Anemia or its twin Myelodysplastic Syndrome (MDS).

Here is a journal entry from Friday, December 7, 2001:

It is now 11 months since I was initially diagnosed with a Bone Marrow Disorder. I met another patient of Dr. Kirshner's today.

He has non-Hodgkin's lymphoma (Non-Hodgkin's lymphomas are a type of cancer of the lymphatic system. There are two main types of lymphoma: one is called Hodgkin's disease (named after Dr Hodgkin, who first described it) and the other is called non-Hodgkin's lymphoma. There are about 20 different types of non-Hodgkin's lymphoma.)

He has been battling the illness for about 5 yrs. and has experienced many highs and lows of remission, re-occurrence, chemotherapy, clinical trials, etc. We had a long discussion about the huge increase in immune related disorders in people of our generation (he is 54 - looks older than me which I am sure is a function of how much longer he has been battling the illness -

He has also concluded that increased toxins in our environment has played a large role in the increase in cancers and other diseases affecting our generation - he read (dr. Samuel Epstein, University of Illinois) that over 75,000 new chemicals have been introduced into the environment since World War II and only 10 % have been tested for their impact on the human organism! Our environment is literally killing us!

Like Mindy who started this chapter, I also led a pretty aggressive life style, never stopping to smell the roses. I ran from one thing to the next, played the music loud and ate at least three meals a day at McDonald's, Taco Bell, Wendy's, KFC and Burger King. My idea of a well-balanced meal was a "Number Six" from Mickey D's. Would you care to upsize that sir for only 29 cents?

Was there any other way to eat? In my past life, vegetables were something that old people grew in their gardens and sold to older people from their roadside stands. Today I had oatmeal for breakfast; rutabagas, cabbage and carrots for lunch; and romaine lettuce, organic brown rice and whole red beans for dinner.

My personal "Journey to Wellness" has been a long one and is now based primarily on eating mostly things that grow naturally in the ground rather than get ground up and processed into plastic tasting fast food.

Chapter 21

On the Merry Go Round

Will This Ever Stop?

Sunday, Nov 4th - Back on the merry go round with a new spin - Got up early, showered and got ready for church then suddenly got severe chills followed by fever up to 103 and spent nearly the whole day fighting it. Sue wanted me to go to ER, I refused and spent the day alternately freezing and roasting in bed.

Monday, Nov 5th - Felt better, showered etc. and went to scheduled visit with Dr. K. - WHAM, 8:30 AM Shaking chills so bad could not hold the phone to call Sue. Transferred via ambulance to CGH. Spent several hours on the 3rd floor (only room available on short notice) getting stable (on oxygen, IV, Tylenol and antibiotics) and then transferred to 469. Rest of the day getting meds and had another episode that night I think - Had about 5-6 but then kind of ran together after a while.

This episode scared the heck out of me – the first time I actually felt frightened. I could not control the shakes and almost went into convulsions at least 3 times where I was about to bite my tongue etc. – I was a lovely experience! Dr. K says it appears to be some kind of bacteria and they will know more after some testing is completed. They took cultures from line and arm and also a CBC to check blood levels.

I experienced a second episode of the shakes for Sue's benefit late in the afternoon and she spent the night with me.

Tuesday, Nov 6th - Early AM severe shaking session. Okay, let's get to work on this one - Two units of blood, 5 pack of platelets, Vancomycin, Cephapime and Saline all day and night. A slave to the IV pole again. Preliminary results confirm bacteria but they still aren't sure what type. Jeff the Elder will check back tomorrow. Sue's sister, Kathy, one of my strongest supporters, spent the next day with me. I provided another late afternoon shaking performance for Kathy and Pastor Darrin. Kathy looked worried so that was a cause for alarm since she sees this stuff all the time as a neo natal intensive care nurse. Melissa spent the night and mercifully there were no additional shaking sessions.

Wednesday, Nov 7th - I greeted the day with yet another shaking session. Dr. Brody (Infection control staff doctor changed the antibiotic mix a bit – took me off the Vancomycin and added something I don't remember) I experienced a sharp pain at my catheter site so they again changed the dressing and did another culture.

Melanie and Fred arrive early Thursday AM after driving all night. Oh, oh this is getting serious. I put on a special matinee performance for them about 2:00 PM.

Dr. K took one look about 4:30 and said, "This is what we call in medicine, a no brainer – the catheter has to go." He had been trying to save it since it was an instrumental tool in my treatment, but the infection continued to worsen, so he scheduled immediate surgery. Dr. Congelli arrived at my room about 8:00 PM gave me a little morphine and Lydocaine, and by 8:30 PM, my old friend Bernie the Hick Man was history.

Bernie saved me from approximately 500 needle sticks so he was a good friend - So long Bernie. It's back to getting needle sticks for Bubba. One of them bruised my arm reminiscent of the first Rochester experience. I have a black bruise about 2" by 4" under my left arm from an IV poke!

Thursday, Nov 8th - Dr K. 10:00 AM "You have septicemia, negative gram rod very serious blood infection that needs to be addressed right away." We will put you back on the vanko immediately. Carol actually stole someone else's dose and it was being delivered via IV drip about 15 minutes after the order was given (normally even a stat takes at least an hour).

Dr Brody later confirmed that I actually had two separate bacterial infections and would receive both Vanko and Cephapime, another very strong antibiotic. They will watch it closely for another day or two and then I will be placed on an oral antibiotic and sent home. Glory Hallelujah! No shakes on Thursday!

Friday, Nov 9th - Released at 10:00 AM with oral SMZ-TMP DS Tabs (Sulfamethoxazole) Known to cause Aplastic Anemia - Now that's interesting! This one sounds like a real winner, but have to get the bacteria under control or it will kill me. Nice choices I have. Speaking of choices:

I am now very concerned about the short duration between transfusions - blood was less than a week and platelets were only 4 days - and they did not respond well at all. I will likely need either or both again early next week. The bacteria episode also is making me seriously reconsider the decision to wait for a BMT until after the holidays. I may not have that long at this rate.

I have witnessed via newsgroups how quickly people can be taken by one of these infections and I don't want to go that way. I sent an email off to Lucy inquiring as to how quickly they could arrange the BMT if I decided to turn up the timetable. We agreed to watch counts this week and probably make an ultimate decision shortly.

To complicate things, we sold our house tonight! Accepted an offer about 7:00 PM on Friday. This will at least stop the financial bleeding. If only it were that as easy to stop my real bleeding!

Chapter 22

My Awakening

Holistic Healing Introduced

He was born in the summer of his twenty-seventh year

Coming home to a place he'd never been before
He left yesterday behind him

You might say he was born again
You might say he found the key to every door
John Denver, Rocky Mountain High

"If you are not going to adhere to the program and do what you are supposed to do, then we did throw the $20,000 away." Sue Lande July 2001

It was well after we had been to the Environmental Health Center in Dallas (EHCD), and I was grumbling about how I had wasted $20,000 of our hard earned money. It had become apparent that Sue's insurance company was not going to pay for this "alternative and experimental" approach and I was seriously considering a Matched Unrelated Donor (MUD) Bone Marrow Transplant (BMT). A BMT is a radical, life threatening procedure, but I wanted this nightmare over NOW and I was willing to take the chance.

I was angry, losing hope and much of my anger was wrongfully directed at what ultimately became my life saving approach. Sue stopped me and after collecting her thoughts, expressed the words that turned my life around: "If you are not going to adhere to the program and do what you are supposed to do, then we did throw the $20,000 away."

We had a very heated discussion about what had been done and not done. I was doing the program prescribed by Dr. Rea of the EHCD in a half-hearted manner and was not yet a true believer. I was still looking for the miracle cure from conventional medicine.

She then said, "You can choose to believe or do what you want, but I resent the fact that you are bad mouthing environmental medicine. I have been researching it for over fifteen years and believe with every fiber of my being that if you would follow the environmental approach; you can beat just about any illness out there - including Aplastic Anemia.

But you can't do it half-assed, you have to do what they say and stay with it for more than a couple of days. You DID NOT do it like they said to do it. As usual, you did it in your "get it done quickly" approach. This is going to take time and you need to change your attitude, buster!"

When Sue ends a statement with "buster" I know two things; she means business and she loves me with her whole heart.

As a Registered Nurse, Sue has been studying Environmental Illness for well over 20 years. She has seen firsthand the differences between conventional drugs oriented treatments and more natural approaches for herself, our daughter and many others.

It has taken me a long time to accept what she has been trying to explain to me, but I am becoming a believer in the philosophy that big Pharmaceutical companies manipulate our attitude towards healing in the same fashion that the tobacco industry lures children into smoking.

Most MD's freely admit that they know very little about natural approaches to healing (they do no teach it in medical school) and in fact are most often only treating symptoms.

After months of being subjected to the conventional and destructive treatments prescribed by conventional wisdom and getting worse by the day, Sue finally convinced me that we had to try something new. I had been in and out of hospitals for over a year and was now in a position where lifting my head off the pillow was a major effort.

Since being diagnosed with Aplastic Anemia in January of 2001, the conventional treatments did nothing but make me sicker. I was on steroids, Cyclosporine, ATG and a host of other meds designed to treat the side effects of the former.

I felt lousy, developed arthritis, had severe joint pain, diarrhea, headaches, cramps and all kinds of other minor symptoms. Since completely dropping these meds, I feel much better and although my counts remain the same, I am hopeful that I am finally taking charge of my situation.

According to Dr. Weill (http://www.drweill.com/Immunity), "your immune system is your interface with the environment. A healthy immune system is the cornerstone of good general health."

He further explains that if you pay attention to the messages your body is sending you through your immune system you can avoid the cancers and other illnesses caused by a malfunctioning immune system. It is usually not that your immune system does not work, but that after sending you messages for so long it finally gives up and can no longer function properly.

Diseases like Aplastic Anemia, MDS, many forms of cancers and so many other are "Autoimmune Disorders in which the immune system attacks the body's own tissues.

Dr. Weill states, "The immune system is hard to understand for several reasons. First of all, it was not recognized as a functional unit of the body until recent years. It is a sobering fact of modern medical history that doctors labeled many of the organs of the immune system "functionless" throughout most of this century, giving surgeons license to remove them with abandon.

The medical profession has removed or destroyed countless tonsils, adenoids, appendixes, thymus glands, and spleens in the belief that these structures were useless, not worth the space they occupied. Second, the components of the immune system do not hang together in any neat arrangement that makes it easy to picture the whole, as we can picture the digestive system or the vascular system. Finally, the operations of the immune system are immensely intricate.

The immune system comprises the tonsils and adenoids, the thymus gland, the lymph nodes throughout the body, the bone marrow, the circulating white blood cells and other cells that leave blood vessels and migrate through tissues and the lymphatic circulation, the spleen, the appendix, and patches of lymphoid tissue in the intestinal tract.

The essential job of this system is to distinguish self from not self, to recognize and take appropriate action against any materials that ought not to be in the body, including abnormal and damaged components. For example, it can seek out and destroy disease germs and cells infected by germs, as well as recognize and destroy tumor cells. In deciding what belongs in the body and what does not, the immune system pays particular attention to details of protein chemistry, because of all the molecules that make up living organisms, proteins are the most distinctive and the most specialized.

As an example of the importance on just one of these organs involve in the immune system, read the following excerpt from http://boobboutique.com, a site dedicated to healing breast cancer:

"The tonsils are an integral part of the body's immune system and lymph system playing an important role in detoxifying the body from impurities and toxins. Many people unknowingly have chronic tonsillitis promoted by a steady stream of toxins produced by infected teeth or by chronically infected paranasal sinuses. These toxins tend to flow through the tonsils via the lymphatic system. At first, the tonsils simply regenerate their tissues after exposure to toxins; increasingly, however, the destroyed tonsil tissue is replaced by inactive scar tissue. The person no longer feels pain or sensation in the tonsils, which often appear superficially healthy.

German physician and researcher Joseph Issels, MD, found upon removing degenerated tonsils, that they were surrounded by a thick, callous capsule which required a sharp instrument to pierce. Upon excising the capsule, Dr. Issels and his colleagues typically found 'multiple small abscesses as well as cherry-sized cysts filled with fluid or thickened pus. The tonsillar tissue was spongy, mushy and had a carcass-like smell.' What is important here is that two-thirds of Dr. Issels' cancer patients had degenerative atrophic tonsils, a fact, which highlights yet another source of toxicity which when combined with other factors could lead to cancer growth. A corollary German study revealed that 85% of patients examined had infected tonsils and that the resulting abscesses had drained into the bloodstream, further toxifying the blood."

Like the nervous system, the immune system is capable of learning. It analyzes its experiences, remembers them, and passes them on to future generations of cells.

Dr. Weill provides excellent information on how to avoid autoimmune disorders on his website. He discusses the causes for the malfunctions and what can be done to avoid them in the first place. He also cautions to avoid the use of steroids, antibiotics and blood transfusions (unfortunately those of us with blood disorders often have no choice until our counts stabilize.)

Like Dr. Rogers and Dr. Rea, Dr. Weill also stresses the importance of a healthy vegetable based diet, avoiding exposure to chemicals and radiation and the importance of hygiene in avoiding the illnesses.

After reading the 100 Days by David Biro and finally seeing the terrible side effects of BMT in real people I was very reluctant to subject myself to this strategy. Instead, I decided to exhaust all other alternatives.

To understand what brought us to this point, we need to explain more about Aplastic Anemia. What does it do to a patient and what are the conventional means of treating it and similar illnesses.

"The doctor of the future will give no medicine but will interest his patients in the care of the human frame, in diet, and in the cause and prevention of disease"
Thomas A. Edison

Chapter 23

The Immune System

How it Works

The immune system is one of the most complex systems of the human body and we are just now beginning to understand how important it is to our health. Doctors randomly removed adenoids, tonsils, spleens and other components of the immune system because they did not understand the functions until very recently.

Researchers still have much to learn about this critical bodily function and breakthrough research is being done every day.

The immune system is the group of organs shown in the diagram below from the National Institute of Allergy and Infectious Diseases Web Site considered to be the body's first line of defense. These cells are very specialized and even have their own circulatory system separate from but working in harmony with blood vessels

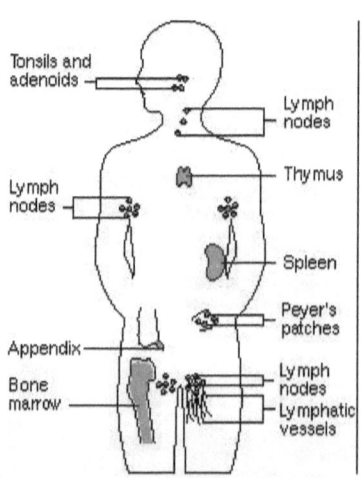

All of the organs work together to clear infection from the body and prevent disease. The organs of the immune system are often referred to as the lymphoid organs.

The lymphatic vessels and lymph nodes carry a fluid called lymph. Lymph is primarily composed of white blood cells, mostly lymphocytes.

The lymphatic system circulates throughout most of the body very similar to blood vessels, but most people don't even know they have a lymphatic system. The system also includes the spleen, which is located upper left of the abdomen. The spleen is a very important component of the entire system, yet is still randomly removed by many surgeons. It serves as a collection point or gathering place for the system cells confront foreign microbes.

Other components of immune system include the bone marrow, thymus, tonsils, adenoids, Peyer's patches, and the appendix. These organs are actually collections of lymph tissues.

Both immune cells and foreign molecules enter the lymph nodes through the skin and via blood vessels or lymphatic vessels. Once they exit the lymphatic system, they return to the bloodstream and are transported to tissues throughout the body, where they are responsible for seeking out foreign antigens.

The bone marrow is actually the largest organ in the body and is responsible for producing many of the cells in our body. The marrow is a spongy tissue found in the center of the large bones including the femur and pelvis. The bone marrow produces pluripotent stem cells that, through a process called mitosis or cell division, generate all the blood cells. The cells are later differentiated and the immune system is most concerned with the cells called lymphocytes.

There are two types of lymphocytes; B cells, which actually mature in the bone marrow, and T cells, which mature in the thymus. The thymus is a tiny organ located behind upper part of your chest bone. It is very active pre puberty but then shrinks in size and is believed to cease functioning completely over time.

The B-lymphocytes are responsible for identifying and marking foreign antibodies and the T-lymphocytes carry out the actual destruction process. This cell marking and destruction process is very involved and in AA, MDS and other autoimmune disorders the process breaks down. For reasons that are still unclear, cells are sometimes incorrectly marked, others are not allowed to mature properly and still others that should be marked for destruction are not. The immune system is said to be out of balance.

The immune system can also become overburdened over time when we ignore the symptoms of rashes, allergic reactions, constipation and other warning signs. These warning signs are our body's way of trying to tell us something is wrong. If we ignore the symptoms, they often get worse and as in my case, escalate to a point that we are forced to take action or die.

The immune system includes a remarkably complex series of chain reactions that, if interrupted or damaged, can have serious consequences. The full discussion about the immune system is available at http://www.niaid.nih.gov/final/immun/immun.htm.

My regimen is designed to rebalance the immune system, and I am continually trying to learn more about how the cells are marked, why they are marked, what can be done to grown healthy cells and prevent their destruction. I have chosen to do this without the intervention of drugs, vitamins or supplements.

Everything I do is now based on a belief that our bodies will function better if we extract the nutrients we need from natural sources.

Chapter 24

Detoxing & Nutrition

A Winning Combination

"If you don't take care of your body, where will you live?"

Aaron Goode, 10 from the preface to Dr. Koop's Self Care Advisor

Our health depends on the immune system, digestive system and elimination system all working together in harmony to prevent disease, provide nourishment and eliminate waste products from our body.

Since the advent of my illness, I have read hundreds of books about the workings of the human body and the various illnesses with which we are confronted. It has been frustrating to see how many books portend to be about healing the body while completely ignoring the immune system and the importance of good nutrition.

Doctors and other medical professionals write the large majority of these books. They prescribe drugs to mask specific symptoms with little regard for the whole individual. This practice actually works against us and exposes us to even more harmful toxins than the hundreds already in our environment.

Two of the best resources I found for developing a sound nutrition plan are The Prescription for Nutritional Healing by Phyllis A. and James F. Balch and Optimal Nutrition for Optimal Health by Thomas E. Levy, M.D.

Dr. Levy states in his introduction, "when the toxic challenges finally overwhelm the immune system, disease will inevitably result. Furthermore, such a disease will also tend to become rapidly entrenched and chronic, since the compromised immune system rarely gets an opportunity to favorably respond to the practice of optimal nutrition along with the removal of toxicity. Rather, such an immune system is usually asked to recover in the face of unchanged toxicity and chronically poor nutrition."

Long before I understood the role of the immune system, I was fortunate enough to begin detoxifying my body at the Environmental Health Center and adapt many of the procedures outlined in the books by Dr. Sherry Rogers.

I continue this process on a regular basis and am convinced that this "detoxing" and good nutrition have been the dual cornerstones for my recovery. Sue and Jeff the Elder saved my life. Sue, Dr. Rea and Dr. Rogers are helping me return to normal.

Good nutrition involves much more than simply changing your diet. To help your body heal itself, you need an understanding of how your digestive system and immune system work in concert to allow for the proper assimilation of nutrients, and rid your body of toxic wastes.

To begin, think of your digestive system as a series of cascading food processors each one with a slightly different function. Place the processors on your kitchen counter and ramp them so they ultimately empty into your garbage disposal. If you don't have a garbage disposal you'll have to use your imagination a little more than the rest of us.

Each processor has a little faucet on the bottom that connects to a piece of plastic tubing connected to the top of the next processor (Got the picture?)*

Now give your processors some labels - say Mouth, Stomach, Small Intestine, Liver, Large Intestine and Colon. Now mix up several different colored jars of water and label them Enzymes One, Two, Three and Four (They have fancy scientific names but I can' remember which one does what so let's just keep things simple.)

Finally, tape a big sign with the words "My Digestive System" on your cupboard door and put some relaxing music in your CD player.

Turn on the CD player for relaxation. Try not to drive while you are using your digestive system because it really stresses everyone out. Drop a bite-sized piece of apple into the processor labeled Mouth. Let it just sit there for a minute and see if it will flow into the stomach without some help. Go ahead and swallow it whole (push it through the tubing to the stomach). If your setup is like mine, you probably broke the tubing and will have to buy some more. Maybe you can pick up an antacid or two to see if that helps!

Okay, now let's be a little kinder to our little digestive system.

Drop in the apple and spin it on puree for about sixty seconds. Add some liquid enzymes and then open the faucet to the Stomach – Amazing how the first step in the process can do so much!

You can aid the digestion process immensely by reducing the initial size of a food portion as much as possible. Try forcing progressively smaller bits through your tubing and observe the results. (Hey, you're a scientist!) The smaller the bits, the easier it will be for the other components of your system to fulfill their respective roles.

Your teeth become processing blades by chopping the apple into progressively smaller bits. This chewing or chopping step is perhaps the most critical step in the whole process (assuming of course you are eating an organically grown apple and not an apple pie from Mickey D's).

Most nutritionists advise us to chew a food particle at least twenty times before swallowing. The more surface area of the apple you can expose to the digestive enzymes in your mouth and later processors, the better off you will be. And, the longer you chew the less you eat and the better your clothes will fit.

Your body actually pours in the various enzymes all the way along the digestive tract. Each one has a separate function, from breaking down protein into various nutrients to regulating the flow of the particles through the system and separating out waste products.

If you push your food through too quickly all sorts of nasty things can happen like "acid reflux", or leaky gut or whatever fancy term Madison Avenue may come up with next week. Maybe you should take a little purple pill and wash it down with a 32-ounce soda (soda does a great job of neutralizing the effectiveness of enzymes) – or, you could slow down, take smaller bites and chew, chew, chew.

Assuming your apple has now been pureed, it should easily flow through the first set of tubing (did we label that esophagus?) into the next processor (stomach).

Once your pureed solution reaches the stomach, the digestive process is in full swing. Your nervous system alerted your stomach that food was on the way and it (your stomach) released some Enzyme number two to begin the sorting process. (If you've ever done laundry, I guess it's like sorting out the whites, colors and dark clothes – I never used to do that, but now that Sue is bringing home the bacon, I have to learn about that stuff)

So, we toss the clothes, I mean food into the stomach and it churns around like your washing machine continuing the chewing process.

Let's see now – proteins and nutrients go in this pile, sugar and red dye #5 and all the polymonosodium carbonated unpronounceable can go right out the back door (the longer they hang around, the more harm they can do), and lets emulsify (liquefy) the rest.

The stomach continues to chew the food (put your blender on slow) and controls how quickly the food mass is released to the small intestine. It also accepts input (oops, that's my computer background) from the liver and gall bladder for the emulsification (washing machine function).

Leave the faucet on your stomach processor partially open all day so small amounts of the food mass can be released to the small intestine. Once in the small intestine, the food is broken down into vitamins, nutrients and amino acids for absorption. The small intestine actually delivers the nutrients to the liver automatically (no faucet required) and the liver decides (you didn't know the liver was so important did you?) what goes where. Keep throwing beer and other nasty stuff at it and eventually it will shut down, become clogged and you'll need a new processor (a liver transplant?).

Once the small intestine and liver have completed their assignments, whatever is left (mostly liquid and waste products is released (open the faucet on your small intestine processor) to the large intestine.

Once in the Large Intestine Processor, and depending on how much junk you have ingested, the food mass can hang around for a few hours. The longer it hangs around, the worse it gets. Dead flesh stuff can actually bind itself to the walls of the intestine and build up over time.

I recommend you periodically flush this processor out with some coffee or some other cleansing agent. (See the chapter on detoxifying your body or pick up a copy of Dr. Sherry Rogers's book "Wellness Against all Odds," or check out the fasting procedure described later on in this chapter.

Oh, by the way, Dr. Levy says you should even chew eggs and Jell-O because you don't want any lumpy stuff getting to the stomach – it causes indigestion or worse just passes it on to the waste station without extracting any nutrients. (All that work of cracking the eggs, frying them up in a pan, tossing in some broccoli for color and you may as well have just tossed them in the disposal).

The rest of your body, including the immune system, depends on the digestive system for the passing of nutrients. If the nutrients never get passed because you digestive system is clogged or malfunctioning, then everything eventually breaks down.

Not only can it bog down and function poorly, if the toxins are allowed to build up in your system over a long period of time, they can cause significant long-term damage. Let's say like, leaving the food to rot in the food processor and going away on vacation.

Not only does the whole house stink when you return, you will likely have attracted all sorts of mean and nasty critters while you were away. Well, guess what, that's what happens to your immune system.

As the toxins build up, they begin to rot out your insides, your whole system gets out of balance, cancer and other nasty things start and before you know it, you are in big trouble. All because you did not feed your body the proper kinds of foods and take the time to do little things like chew your food instead of swallowing it whole.

Signing off from the kitchen,

Chef Charisse

* * * * *

*If you prefer the more scientific explanation of this whole process, please locate a copy of "Optimal Nutrition for Optimal Health."

As must be obvious by now, I can become easily confused in the kitchen and I am not a doctor - and this is certainly no joking matter, - but I am an amateur plumber (I have installed at least six bathrooms and cleaned the pipes in more than I care to remember) so I understand the importance of a healthy, well-functioning drainage system. So let's consider our body's elimination system as a drainage system.

If you've never been behind the walls of your house, you probably don't realize the set of pipes that run from your kitchen sink (oh, my God, Mildred he even got the kitchen sink in his book) out to the street and on to the disposal plant. The pipes get progressively larger as you move from a 1 ¼ " sink trap to the 3" main stack and then out to the street (or cesspool if you have your own system) to connect with the larger mainlines.

What is interesting for our discussion is how if there is a serious clog in the main stack (we could call that the colon I suppose?), it doesn't much matter how much your work on the trap in your kitchen sink. Your entire system will simply get more sluggish as you continue to force more stuff down the drain. Eventually it will plug up so badly, that you'll have to access your main stack "cleanout" or if you don't know what that is, call your Rotor Rooter man and have him clean out your entire system.

Now, in the case of our elimination system, after years of a poor diet, lack of exercise and neglect, our colon becomes caked with debris and toxins build up in the liver and other organs. Just as you may need to flush out your plumbing system with Drain-o or Liquid Plumber occasionally, so too should you clean out your internal drainage system (but please, don't use the plumbing liquids.)

In her book, Wellness against All Odds, Dr. Rogers explains the importance of this regular detoxification process in conjunction with the other elements of a wellness plan:

"One of the things that impressed me in watching people improve cancers, chemical sensitivity and other conditions with the coffee enemas is the steadiness with which it must be done. It must be a daily routine and for weeks on end there may be no improvement and then suddenly everything clicks in and improvement can be appreciated.

For some, it takes months before the body rallies. It is the steadiness however, that is so important and it is a steadiness of a total load program which includes the correct diet, enzymes, hormones, juicing, prescribed nutrients, periodic bowel cleanse and flushing, attention to ones' spirituality, and environmental controls. These all constitute an important part of the total load whenever coffee enemas are used. They should not be used in isolation or alone without a total program. And above all, they should be done with good nutrient supplementation and periodic checking of nutrient levels."

The Coffee Enema for Detoxifying the Liver*

What you will need:

1. Enema bag – Most pharmacies have or can get them

2. A bunch of old towels
3. Folgers regular grind coffee
4. Pure spring water or steam distilled water
5. Small bottle of organic oil or vitamin E capsules

The Procedure

1. Boil 4 tablespoons of coffee in 1 quart (4 cups) of water for at least 10 minutes and allow to cool to room temperature

2. Hang the enema bag around waist height and fill it ½ the solution (1 pint or 2 cups) Make sure the clamp is secure if not you will be glad I suggested the towels

3.   Place an old towel in the bathtub (saves mess later) and assume the position best described by Phyllis Balch in Prescription for Natural Healing (on your knees with head down, rear up)

4.   Lubricate the tip with organic oil or the liquid from a vitamin E capsule and gently insert the enema tube (you may want to find a softer tip if you can)
5.   Slowly release the clamp and allow the liquid to flow. I usually release for a count of 6 and then stop for a count of 20 or 30
6.   Lie on your first right side and retain the liquid for at least 5-10 minutes (this may be difficult at first but will become easier later) and then evacuate
7.   Repeat

I do this at least five days per week and credit it as one of the keys to my success.

*This has been compiled from multiple sources and I believe it to be safe, but I am not a doctor and I caution you to consult with a nutritionist or medical professional before implementing this or any other elements of my program. I may error on the side of too much detail, but hopefully this will same you some time as you develop your own plan.

Almost two years after my diagnosis and while reading the Prescription for Nutritional Healing, I discovered the concept of a regular fast and decided to also give this a try. The results were amazing and I am surprised this concept has not received more attention from other sources. Even in the Balch book it is buried at the end.

According to the Balch's, the fasting process, when used in conjunction with lemon juice and coffee enemas, reduces the workload on the immune system and gives all your organs a much needed rest from the toxin removal chores.

The procedure they recommend and what I followed was as follows:

1.	Two days before beginning the true fast, eat only raw organic vegetables
2.	On day three, drink only organic juices, herbal teas and at least 8 glasses of pure water
3.	Drink two or three cups or juiced or broth boiled of cabbage, carrots, alfalfa sprouts, celery, beets, garlic and onion. Save the actual vegetables for eating later.
4.	Do a daily coffee enema and a daily lemon juice enema – they say to use 3 lemons in 2 quarts of water and use the same process as described above except there is more frequent expelling and when you can lay on your left side and massage your colon and abdomen.

As mentioned, this simple process worked wonders for me. I was surprisingly not hungry once I got into it and felt like my whole body had been cleansed.

In the next chapter, I will summarize my understanding of Dr's Rogers, Balch, Rea, Gerson and several others. I encourage you to read as many of these books as you can and develop your own plan, but here then is my synopsis.

Chapter 25

Nutritional Healing

A Brief History

Many components of the healing process that I adopted have been around since time began, but it was not until about 1950 that the medical community of the 20th century began to understand the natural healing process as it related to modern cancers and other toxic related disorders.

Unfortunately one of the downsides of our 21st century is our propensity for newer, better and faster. We want a pill that will immediately make a headache go away, never mind that the headache may be trying to tell us something is wrong with our body or we are consuming something that is not good for us.

We are constantly bombarded with the latest magic pill guaranteed to stifle the sneeze, stop the headache, or stop the runny nose when in essence every one of these actions is our body attempting to alert us to the dangers of the environment and the abuses being hurtled at us from every corner.

So in our approach to healing our bodies is it any wonder that we expect to pop a pill and have all our troubles go away?

In developing my Personal Wellness Plan, I borrowed from many disciplines and sources. Perhaps the best way of explaining how I arrived at what I am doing today is to share many of my readings.

* * * * *

The Prescription for Nutritional Healing lists six categories of Alternative Cancer Therapies:

- Biologic and Pharmacologic
- Herbal
- Immunologic
- Metabolic
- Mind-Body
- Nutritional

Without realizing it at the time, my approach primarily borrows from Immunologic as espoused by Dr. Josef Issels; Metabolic, first introduced by Dr. Max Gerson and Nutritional as practiced by Dr. Sherry Rogers and many others. I have also tried some Mind-Body techniques including visualization. I am essentially treating both the body and the disciplines as a whole rather than trying any single approach.

Many of today's alternative and holistic approaches appear to have evolved from the work done by Dr. Max Gerson in the 1950's and by the 1954 Nobel Chemist, Linus Pauling in the 60's and 70's.

Doctor Josef Issels

Source: http://www.issels.org/

"Josef M. Issels, MD, has become internationally known for his remarkable rate of complete long-term remissions of "incurable cancers" in patients who had exhausted all standard treatments, such as advanced cancers of the breast, uterus, prostate, colon, liver, lung, brain, sarcomas, lymphomas, and leukemia.

After completion of the Issels Treatment, these patients remained cancer free for up to 45 years, leading normal healthy lives. The Issels Treatment also significantly reduced the incidence of recurrent cancer after surgery, radiation, and chemotherapy, thereby considerably improving cure rates.

The Issels Treatment was able to reverse chronic degenerative diseases such as arthritis, lupus, Grave's disease, Sjoegren's syndrome, asthma, etc.

According to the concept that cancer starts as a locally confined growth, all measures concentrated on the tumor alone seem causal and exhaustive.

Treating the tumor alone is not treating the condition that is producing it: the underlying malignant disease. Consequently, there is a high rate of relapse.

According to the holistic concept, however, cancer is considered a systemic disease from the onset and the tumor as its late stage symptom."

Gerson Therapy for Cancer and Other Illnesses

Source: http://www.gerson.org/

Albert Schweitzer labeled Dr. Gerson "a genius of medicine."

"The Gerson Therapy is a powerful, natural treatment that boosts your body's own immune system to heal cancer, arthritis, heart disease, allergies, and many other degenerative diseases. One aspect of the Gerson Therapy that sets it apart from most other treatment methods is its all-encompassing nature. An abundance of nutrients from thirteen fresh, organic juices are consumed every day, providing your body with a super dose of enzymes, minerals and nutrients. These substances then break down diseased tissue in the body, while enemas aid in eliminating the lifelong buildup of toxins from the liver.

With its whole-body approach to healing, the Gerson Therapy naturally reactivates your body's magnificent ability to heal itself - with no damaging side effects. Over 200 articles in respected medical literature, and thousands of people cured of their "incurable" diseases document the Gerson Therapy's effectiveness. The Gerson Therapy is one of the few treatments to have a 60-year history of success.

The Gerson Therapy is a state of the art, contemporary, holistic and natural treatment which utilizes the body's own healing mechanism in the treatment and cure of chronic debilitating illness. When it was introduced to the world by Max Gerson, M.D., the dietary therapy was so far ahead of its time that there were almost no rationales available in the scientific literature to explain how it could produce cures in chronic as well as infectious diseases.

Most therapies, conventional or alternative treat only the individual symptoms while ignoring what is ultimately causing the disease. The reason the Gerson Therapy is effective with so many different ailments is because it restores the body's incredible ability to heal itself. Rather than treating only the symptoms of a particular disease, the Gerson Therapy treats the cause of the disease itself. Although we feel the Gerson Therapy is the most comprehensive treatment for disease, we don't claim it will cure everything or everyone."

Linus Pauling – Linus Pauling Institute

Source: http://lpi.oregonstate.edu/

Winner of the 1954 Nobel Prize for Chemistry

"The Linus Pauling Institute functions from the basic premise that an optimum diet is the key to optimum health. Our mission is to determine the function and role of micronutrients, vitamins, and phytochemicals in promoting optimum health and preventing and treating disease; to determine the role of oxidative and nutritive stress and antioxidants in human health and disease; and to advance knowledge in areas that were of interest to Linus Pauling through research and educational activities.

Major areas of research in the Institute encompass heart disease, cancer, aging, neurodegenerative diseases, immune dysfunction and disease caused by exposure to toxins. Specific laboratories address antioxidants and vascular biology; vitamin E metabolism and biological activity; colon cancer and cancer chemoprevention by phytochemicals; the role of nitric oxide and oxidative stress in neurodegenerative diseases, such as ALS (Lou Gehrig's disease); and the role of oxidative stress and mitochondrial dysfunction in the aging process.

Linus Pauling is often considered the founding father of molecular biology, which has transformed the biological sciences and medicine and provided the base for biotechnology.

Popular books in which he detailed his nutritional recommendations are Vitamin C and the Common Cold, Cancer and Vitamin C (with Ewan Cameron, M.D.), and How to Live Longer and Feel Better."

It also seems clear that many of the remedies and approaches have been around for centuries and were practiced by several ancient civilizations including the Chinese, American Indians any many others.

Traditional Chinese Medicine

Source: http://www.healthy.net

What It Does

Chinese medicine is a complete medical system that has diagnosed, treated, and prevented illness for over twenty-three centuries. While it can remedy ailments and alter states of mind, Chinese medicine can also enhance recuperative power, immunity, and the capacity for pleasure, work, and creativity.

How It Thinks

Within Chinese Cosmology, all of creation is born from the marriage of two polar principles, Yin and Yang: Earth and Heaven, winter and summer, night and day, cold and hot, wet and dry, inner and outer, body and mind. Harmony of this union means health, good weather, and good fortune, while disharmony leads to disease, disaster, and bad luck. The strategy of Chinese medicine is to restore harmony.

Each human is seen as a world in miniature, a garden in which doctor and patient together strive to cultivate health. Every person has a unique terrain to be mapped, a resilient yet sensitive ecology to be maintained. Like a gardener uses irrigation and compost to grow robust plants, the doctor uses acupuncture, herbs and food to recover and sustain health.

Other more recent and well-known practitioners of holistic and alternative medicine include Dr. Mercola, Dr. Weill, Dr. Day and many others. I encourage you to read everything you can find and develop your own Personal Wellness Plan. It is time and consuming but well worth the effort. It can save your life!

Chapter 26

Holy Trinity Lutheran Church

A Personal Testimony

"In every cloud, there is a silver lining." Anonymous

For several months prior to my diagnosis, Sue and I had been attending a small rural church in search of a new spiritual home. We raised our kids in another church nearby but since Michelle's illness felt lost. We were angry with God for a number of reasons (I lost both my parents at very young ages and Michelle was diagnosed with a serious illness at thirteen that would forever alter our lives).

After almost ten years, we had come to grips with Michelle's illness and our situation in life. I had started the new business, Sue was happy in her role of School Nurse come Mother Hen to the lost souls in Elementary School. But we knew something was still missing.

Since the kids left home, we had drifted away from church and knew that we were lost spiritually. The pastor of our previous church had retired and we were not comfortable with the new one so in desperation we went back to a small country church in Skaneateles. We visited this one in our original efforts to find a church close to our hometown of Marcellus, but were turned off the by the "hell fire and brimstone" approach of the pastor.

On this visit, however, we found a completely different style of preaching and a young pastor whom we really liked. He has a down to earth style and that unique quality of making everyone feel special – from the old timers to the newly baptized children and as a bonus, our old pastor from St. Michaels was a member and guest preached on occasion.

Pastor Derron has since become a friend and confidant. We were about to join the church when I was first diagnosed and since my spiritual life was in disarray I asked if he would come and see me even though we were not yet members. I remember the visit like it was yesterday.

I completely broke down and cried like a baby. Told him that I really needed to be closer to God and could he help. He listened, counseled and brought me make the inner peace that was lost so many years before.

As a result of joining the church we have also been introduced to many friendly, caring people who have taken a genuine interest in my physical health and our spiritual rebirth. Sue has developed several very close friendships, I joined the choir and we have a church home! So it is true, that there is a silver lining in every cloud.

On a similar subject, I recall asking Sue to get me a cross while I was in Rochester the first time. I had been praying and talking to God about my illness but did not have anything to hold onto. I'm not catholic so I couldn't do rosary beads and I had long ago worn out the "feel good" bead bracelets given to me, so I wanted something to turn over in my hands during the long days in the hospital.

Sue bought me one that had an inscription on it that I had heard before but did not know much about:

"As for me and my house, we will serve the Lord."

It turns out the passage is from the book of Joshua and this was long before our grandson Joshua was even a gleam in his mother's eye. I believe God was telling me that it was not yet my time and the birth of Joshua is his way of telling me that I am still needed here on earth.

Now prominently displayed in Josh's bedroom is the same passage that kept me going when at my worst and the day he was born, May 24, 2002 is the last time I needed a blood transfusion!

"Jesus will save me," My Dad on his deathbed.

Chapter 27

A Resolution to Save My Life

It is the Only Mission

Upon returning from Dallas I was very disillusioned and was beginning to lose hope but decided to give the EHCD and Sherry Rogers approach one more solid effort. When faced with major life challenges (career change, new business, etc.) I would take a very business-like approach, developing a mission statement, and objective and a list of tasks necessary to accomplish my goal.

Even while fighting the illness I tried to remain active in the business and was looking for ways to help save what we had started. Sue remarked that I needed to put all my energy into getting better or it would not matter what happened with anything else. Duh! I decided to take develop a plan for saving my life.

My/Our New Life Resolution April 24, 2002:

My last life-threatening episode at the hands of modern medicine occurred on April 16th, 2002. On April 24th, I resolved to find a better way and my personal holistic approach was launched.

My notes from April 24th started like this:

I will begin with a serious six-month effort to saving my life. I will adhere closely to the EHCD regimen and get myself better. I will disengage from the business and other activities to concentrate on saving my life.

Objective:

Design and implement a diet that will stimulate the growth of healthy red blood cells, white blood cells and platelets. Proof of success will be determined by a RISE in my blood counts from something other than transfusions.

I have always been one to clearly state my goals and design a plan to reach them, so why should this effort be any different. Up until now I had been treating my illness as something that would go away or miraculously take care of itself. I was not treating it seriously and yet continued to grow weaker as time went on. In April of 2002, I finally made getting my health back my number one priority.

I was and am determined to beat this illness and I will try anything and everything in my power. I made a list of my alternatives and weighed the pluses and minuses of each approach. The list included:

- Macrobiotic Diet
- Organic Foods
- Shark Cartilage
- Herbs and Teas
- Dr. Rea Supplements
- Dr. Rogers Supplements
- Cytoxan
- Bone Marrow Transplant

- Rotational Diet
- Biogen
- Alfalfa Greens
- Blood Type Specific Remedies
- Sondra's Magic Potion
- Dr. Gold

The more I researched, the more confused I became. It seemed like there were so many contradictions. I told myself that if I had not seen positive progress by October of 2002, I would go for Cytoxan treatment or maybe even a full BMT because the older I get, the less likely a BMT would be successful.

I spent a lot of time in self-analysis. On reflecting back, one of the things that I found most perplexing was my reluctance to give the alternative strategy a full trial. After all, the conventional treatments were extremely dangerous and toxic. They had almost killed me four times and I really did not have a lot to lose in just giving them a try. I think the reluctance came from a lifelong distrust of anything unconventional.

I was raised in a conventional, mainstream environment. The family doctor was a local hero and the father of one of my best friends. Everyone trusted his judgment and "Dr. Joe" was one the most respected people in the community. It was difficult for me to accept that doctors did not have all the answers. I think I had also had been brain washed into thinking that prescription drugs were the answer to all ailments. At one time I was taking 15 different medications.

The problem was they were not healing me and they were making feel worse. Finally, I seemed to have an innate distrust of the "alternative" approach. It was almost as if I had been conditioned to not believe. I am really not sure where this feeling came from, but it was there

I see this same distrust of the alternative approach in people I talk to and people who visit the website. They listen politely and then blindly accept the recommendations to administer chemotherapy that is potentially far more deadly.

According to Doctors Rogers, Rea, Weill and many others, chemotherapy and steroid use does more harm than good. Antibiotics and other frequently prescribed medications often list Aplastic Anemia as a side effect.

Why is it that we will subject our bodies to these terrible side effects when a properly implemented alternative approach can provide a safer and less destructive result? Since opting out of conventional treatments and into the holistic approach described in the chapter of the same name, I feel stronger, can think again, my blood counts have stabilized and I have hope for a lasting and durable cure.

Perhaps one of my biggest frustrations when I talk to others is their resistance to my approach after I have proven that it works, but then I remember I was the same way and I go back to trying to gently persuade them to at least look at the pluses and minuses of each approach.

From all the research I have been able to find and from my own limited ability to research the outcomes, it appears that Bone Marrow Transplants are only successful about 30 percent of the time. That means that seven out of ten people die within four years of the procedure. I was all set to have a Matched Unrelated Donor (MUD) Bone Marrow Transplant (BMT) at the Bone Marrow Transplant Center in Rochester until I learned that in the past year they had done five procedures and all five people died!

This chart from the National Marrow Donor Program provides further evidence that a Bone Marrow Transplant is a very risky procedure. And these results do not differentiate MUD's from identically matched siblings. I am sure the results are even worse for MUDS.

NMDP Transplant Outcomes for Non-Leukemia

Disease	# Of Transplants	Kaplan-Meier 4-Year Survival*
Severe Aplastic Anemia	288	36% ± 7%
Myelodysplastic & Related Syndromes	578	26% ± 4%
Non-Hodgkin's Lymphoma	201	24% ± 7%
Other Non-Malignant Diseases	438	43% ± 5%

*June 1999 *with 95% Confidence Interval*

It is against my nature to take away someone's hope, but it would seem to me that one would try virtually everything else before dealing with those odds. By the way, the older you get, the more the odds work against you.

With these sobering statistics in hand and after having talked or corresponded with several people who had tried the various approaches listed above, I ultimately decided to develop my own strategy that included the best of several different programs. The strategy is discussed in detail in the chapter on Holistic Medicine, but first let me explain some of the research that led me to my strategy.

Chapter 28

Researching Your Illness

Suggested Process

Since Aplastic Anemia and MDS are such rare illnesses, there is a limited attraction for anyone to do any serious research. The treatments that have been developed were actually developed for other illnesses and have been adapted for use in the treatment of AA and MDS. Most doctors treating the illnesses rely on the research done by the National Institute of Health.

Because it is considered and orphan disease, NIH doesn't even really recognize the illness enough to track progress so we patients are essentially on our own.

After realizing that nobody in the medical or research community was ever going to put any serious effort into finding a lasting cure for Aplastic Anemia, I launched my own research effort. I began by trying to track my belief that AA was somehow a hereditary illness and thought that if I learned more about genetics and DNA that I might discover something that would help.

The fundamental question relative to Aplastic Anemia is, "What can be done to assist the body in the creation of healthy blood cells and/or reversing the destruction process that is preventing these cells from entering the blood stream."

According to the science of immunopathology, the immune system is clearly a "good thing", but like mercenary armies, out of control, it can turn to bite the hand that feeds it and cause damage to the host.

As the most fundamental element of life a DNA molecule is a double helix (strand) consisting of two long strings coiled around one another. The strings are made up of complex nitrogen-bearing chemical compounds called nucleotides. There are four different kinds of nucleotides in DNA, depending on their bases, either adenine, quinine, cytosine, or thymine. Each nucleotide in one string is chemically connected to a corresponding nucleotide in the other string. There may be many thousands of nucleotides in one string, with as many connections to what are like mirror images in the other string of the pair. A gene is a section of a DNA molecule.

Every cell of an individual living thing contains the DNA molecule for that individual. When the cell divides (mitosis), one of the DNA strings goes to the other string to the other cell.

I developed my own set of questions and theories and systematically went about trying to simplify the entire process. I highly recommend you do your own independent research by reading everything you can find and being careful not to skip over something you don't understand the first time. There is an online medical dictionary listed on the home page of aplastic central that was invaluable to me in my efforts.

As previously stated, you are your own best resource in combating your illness but it helps to find a mentor. I enlisted the help of my nephew, Kenton who is a researcher for a pharmaceutical company and is well grounded in cellular biology. We corresponded via email when I was in Texas and by the time I was done, he paid me the supreme complement of telling me I would have made a good scientist.

I found the Internet to be an unbelievable resource in my quest for knowledge. It sometimes took a while to zero in on the information I needed, but eventually by posing the right question on google.com or askjeeves.com and sifting through the responses I was able to find what I needed.

I used my laptop plugged into a phone line so things were sometimes agonizingly slow, but I had plenty of time on my hands while in the Texas condo without Sue. I am a bit of a techno-freak and my toys became very helpful. I have a desktop computer that is my primary link to the outside world and I have the aforementioned laptop computer that I use whenever I am away from home in hospital beds, hotel rooms, etc.

I also have a palmtop with a full-size keyboard that comes in very handy when a laptop is not practical. Using these devices and some handwritten journals (could not use a computer anywhere at EHCD because of the electromagnetic forces being emitted) I was able to build a working knowledge of the various disciplines I needed.

If you have any illness or actually any subject that requires you to develop a better understanding, take advantage of the Internet. It is and continues to be an invaluable resource tool for my efforts. So, with all these tools at my disposal, here is what I have learned.

Beginning at a fairly macro level and believing that my immune system was the primary part of my body that was malfunctioning, I learned that the liver is the key organ in the immune system. It filters the blood and removes harmful bacteria by eliminating impurities into the colon but only if the colon is functioning properly.

The thymus is another organ that is important to people with blood disorders. It is located in the upper interior chest and essentially dictates the health of the immune system. It secretes hormones and produces the specialized white blood cells called T Lymphocytes that control cell mediated immunity. Cell mediated immunity refers to the immune activity that is not controlled by or mediated by antibodies.

The thymus is very active when we are children; building the antibodies we need to combat illnesses throughout our lifetime. When we reach puberty, its role diminishes and it actually shrinks in size.

In The Rebellious Body, it is suggested that we try reviving the role of the thymus by thumping on it for several minutes on a regular basis. It is located an inch below the collar bone in the center of the chest and you simply tap this spot with a rhythmic motion for a few minutes a few times a day.

Since Aplastic Anemia is a condition of bone marrow failure that arises from injury to or abnormal expression of the stem cell and the thymus is instrumental in creating stem cells, it makes sense to me and I try it on a fairly regular basis.

Unfortunately there is really no way of pinpointing any one thing that is working for me, but I am convinced that the combination of my detoxification routine, changing my diet and lifestyle, the antigens as prescribed by the EHCF and my daily sauna/detoxification regimen have been instrumental in me regaining control of my life.

From my research into molecular and cellular biology, I learned that the thyroid produces hormones that are essential to the regulation of metabolism or the rate that cells burn oxygen. These hormones are important in all bodily functions.

I read about "Mitosis" or cell division in an effort to understand what was going wrong with the creation of my cells that would cause them to be improperly marked.

The chart below is worth spending some time with if you want to better understand the terminology associated with cell division. Take a line and follow it like a family tree and many of the terms being used will make more sense. Notice that the left tree is all about red blood cells (erythrocytes), the right side is about platelets (megakaryocytes) and the three lines in the middle all represent different types of white blood cells.

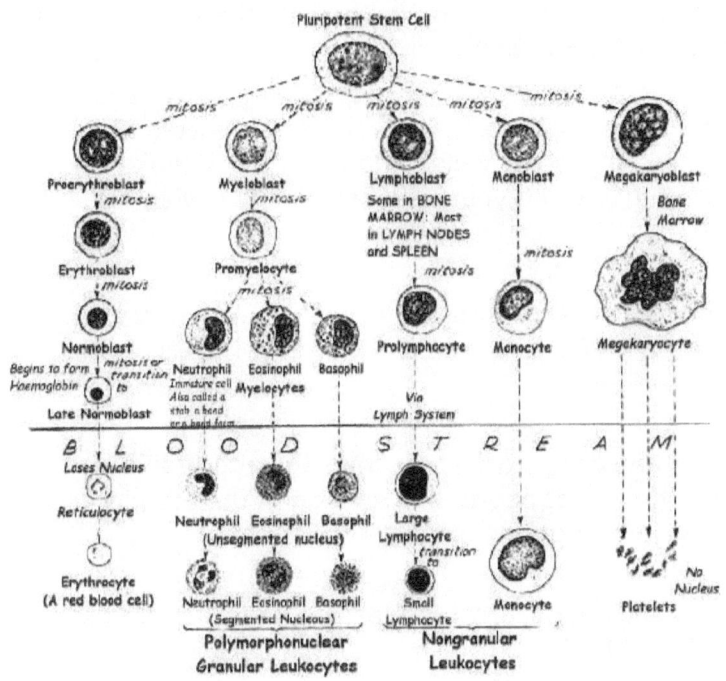

Once I had a better understanding of haematopoeisis (blood cell division), it became easier to understand what point in the process is breaking down in the body of an AA/MDS patient.

For instance, the statement "the granulocytes attack germs in a process called phagocytosis*," makes much more sense when you see where granulocytes are in the tree.

*Phagocytosis, apoptosis and TNF- Tumor Necrosis Factor all refer to the usually normal process of cell destruction.

The granulocytes are sometimes too aggressive and other times not aggressive enough in the marking and destroying of germs and cells.

In my Internet searching I learned that the CD34 marker (CD34 is a transmembrane glycoprotein constitutively expressed on endothelial cells and on hematopoietic stem cells.) is missing or deficient in patients with Aplastic Anemia.

According to Dr. Neil Young of the National Institute of Health "morphologically, the bone marrow is devoid of hematopoietic (blood cell formation) elements, showing largely fat cells. Flow-cytometry shows that the CD34 is diminished."

He continues to say that "this highly O-glycosylated molecule, containing serine and threonine-rich mucin like domains, binds to L-selectin, but its functional capacity in non-lymphatic venules is uncertain. Studies have suggested that CD34 is important in tethering lymphocytes."

The report finishes with "mice deficient in CD34 exhibited no detectable abnormalities in post-surgical leukocyte rolling in cremaster venules. Antibodies blocking L-selectin function reduced rolling in CD34 deficient mice suggesting that CD34 lacks major significance as a ligand for L-selectin. The endothelial ligands for L-selectin are currently unknown.) "

As my own best advocate, I am continuing in these efforts on a regular basis. I am trying to link the NIH report above with the studies that Dr. Rea is conducting. For example, I see that many of my amino acids

(Cystine, threonine and others) are low. Could it be that if these amino acids return to normal levels that my blood levels will follow?

Nobody can give me a clear answer but it is suggested that I begin by taking the additional supplements (Cystine, Arginine and Threonine)

There is a big part of me that is questioning this whole approach. I have now substituted dozens of meds with dozens of vitamins and supplements. Are they really doing anything?

I also read about a theory called "Free Radical Damage." In this theory, the DNA in our cells can supposedly be altered or destroyed by reactive substances in our bodies. When the destroyed DNA is a part of the immune control function, it can result in a specific autoimmune disease.

Just as oxygen outside our bodies can cause iron to rust and is necessary for paper to burn; on the inside, it can be equally destructive. Free radicals are particles that have an unstable molecular structure. They act as scavengers in the body and rob electrons from other molecules to increase their stability.

The particles that are robbed don't function as they should and can be toxic. There are several types of free radicals. Some of the most common have an oxygen base. Free radicals build over time. They are a natural byproduct of our metabolism and immune system functions.

They are a natural component of aging. Stress, pollution, fertilizers, pesticides, prescription drugs, alcohol, electromagnetic radiation, etc. hasten their production. Our bodies have built in controls for free radicals and ways of changing them into neutral substances.

These detoxification mechanisms require specific enzymes to make them function well. If our bodies do not have the vitamins and minerals to make up the enzymes, or if the detoxification mechanism is damaged, perhaps by free radicals, the result is a surplus of free radicals and other toxic substances.

This can also happen if our life style and environment results in our having too many toxins for even a good working system to neutralize. The excess free radicals and other noxious byproducts of a failed detox process roam our bodies and attack our weakest links. These weak links may be due to genetics.

They may be other parts of our immune system that happen to be nearby. Depending on the DNA attacked, the electron grabbing can cause an autoimmune disease.

Theoretically, if a surplus of free radicals is the cause of the disease, reducing the amount of things that promote their production (ex. stress), ingesting substances that reduce the number of free radicals (ex. Vitamin C) and making sure our detoxification mechanisms have sufficient nutrients (eating well) may be part of the cure.

By now, I am thoroughly confused yet even more determined to develop an approach that will work. I now have a better understanding of Dr. Rogers' assertion that most doctors no longer treat the whole person. Because of the complexities of each branch of modern medicine and often by necessity, they become specialists and lose sight of the entire functioning of the body, mind and spirit.

It is with this newfound understanding that I take still another slight detour in my approach and begin to develop a more holistic approach to dealing with my illness. I continue to research at a cellular level, but am approaching my illness and my body in its entirety.

My Research Process for Aplastic Anemia

Here is a copy of the research pages from aplastic central as it existed on March 1, 2003:

I am convinced that there is a way to cure Aplastic Anemia and the answer lies in understanding why and how the immune system decides to attack immature cells. Finding a cure will require the understanding of the various disciplines listed below and I will use this area of the site to store everything I am currently researching.

I will constantly try to put everything into layman's terms. My mission is to simplify, simplify, simplify! People who constantly try to mystify this stuff are exactly like the computer professionals who try to keep people in the dark - the old mushroom theory (keep 'em in the dark and feed 'em shit). Well, I refused to be kept in the dark in the world of data processing and I now refuse to be kept in the dark relative to my disease!

As a starting point, my initial bone marrow aspirate and smears revealed "mildly hyper cellular marrow with mild hyperplasia or erythrocyte series and hypoplasia of megakaryocytes." This means that my marrow has a slightly larger number of cells in a cross section of the marrow than is normal and an abnormal multiplication or increase in the number of normal cells with a lower number of megakaryocytes. Megakaryocytes are the giant polypoid cells (the cells containing the genetic structure or chromosomes necessary for producing additional cells) of bone marrow that gives rise to 3-4,000 platelets each. So in essence, I have a reduced number of the cells necessary to create platelets.

If anyone reading this sees information that is incorrect or misinterpreted, please send me a note of correction. Thanks.

BTW, much of my cursory research while I am traveling will now be at the forum. It's easier to just send my comments there rather than opening and editing the website.

The Disciplines Involved

In addition to the obvious (clinical trials, treatment protocols and survivability), I am trying to understand the following disciplines as they relate to AA:

- Biology
- Immunology
- Immunopathology
- Biochemistry
- Hematology
- Microbiology
- Genetics and DNA Research
- Human Genome Project
- Multiple Chemical Sensitivities
- Alternative Medicines
- Nutrition and Allergies
- Stem Cells
- Pathophysiology

How to Start - The Scientific Method

Above link is a good place to start by understanding how blood cells are produced. Dr. Rea said that the biopsy from Strong said I had no Megakaryocytes (A megakaryocyte is the "progenitor" of platelets - one megakaryocyte produces 4000 platelets) present - That is a serious concern as Megakaryocytes is what produces platelets. No Megakaryocytes, no platelet production! I asked Sharon to send the biopsy results from Strong to EHCD.

Nobody mentioned megakaryocytes to me until Dr. Rea came along. Now I understand that my problem is more at the level of megakaryocytes than it is at the platelet level. If I could keep my body from destroying megakaryocytes, it would then produce platelets? Now that I think about it, Dr. Kirshner talked about "immature platelets" and he must have been referring to megakaryocytes (thank god somebody speaks English).

So now when I read Dr. Young's pathophysiology, it is beginning to make a little more sense. As Richard Laughlin told me a long time ago, the key to understanding what you read is to not let a single word go by that you do not understand. I literally have to look up every word in his report and then look up the words used to define what I looked up before the fog lifts.

I believe that each of these disciplines plays some part in developing a thorough understanding of the autoimmune and blood related illnesses. It is a huge undertaking and I am being bombarded with new terminology in each discipline but I will be attempting to sort it out as I go and this is where it will start.

The scientific method is often divided into steps. This is helpful for putting the method into context, but keep in mind that the key element of the scientific method is testing the hypothesis. In other words, can you prove that you are wrong?

1. Observe the situation
2. Ask a question
3. Turn that question into a testable hypothesis
4. Predict the outcome of your experiment
5. Perform your experiment
6. Analyze the results
7. Evaluate your hypothesis

The Questions and Some Answers

I am beginning to believe that what will be most important in my battle is clearly asking the right questions and then researching the answers, so here are some questions I am working:

1. Is Aplastic Anemia considered an autoimmune disease?

In acquired aplastic anemia, clinical and laboratory observations suggest that this is an autoimmune disease. http://aplasticcentral.org/aplastic_facts.htm

2. How does the immune system relate to the blood system?

Ongoing reading but some fundamentals - At a cellular level, the immune system is charged with remembering microorganisms that are causing problems and develops antigens to destroy these rogue microorganisms. If the blood cells become targets of the immune system (or apoptosis which is programmed death of unnecessary cells), then the blood cells are in trouble because the immune system is very good at what it does - protect the body from microorganisms it doesn't like (It even remembers that you had chicken pox as a kid and if any small pox like microorganisms show up it destroys them)

3. What exactly is happening when the lymphocytes attack the immature platelets and how can I follow that thread to understand the immune system malfunctioning - what is Dr. Rea doing to stimulate platelet growth?

T Lymphocytes are responsible for fighting infections and it appears that in Aplastic Anemia, our lymphocytes have decided that the progenitor cells are an infection? There must be some connection between the fact that I am low in protein and CD34 is a "glycoprotein.

4. Better yet - make sure I understand in detail lymphocytes, CD34 and T cells and apoptosis, etc. and then formulate the questions.

Thanks to Kenton, gaining a much better understanding, but still have a ways to go. Apoptosis is a necessary and natural process the body uses to rid itself of damaged cells or cells that are no longer functioning. Our issue is not really with apoptosis, but with our evolving or precursor blood cells being prematurely marked for destruction.

5. How does environmental illness and Multiple Chemical Sensitivity relate to Aplastic Anemia?

Best guess so far (9/30/01) is that in addition to inheriting a pre-disposition to an autoimmune disease, my body's immune system began to malfunction as a result of being continually exposed to a series of viruses (shingles, meningitis) and toxins (pesticides, mercury, paint, fertilizer, varnishes, molds). If we can isolate the causes by testing what my body may react to, we can prepare and inject antigens to correct the imbalance. At the same time, I do the physical therapy (exercise, sauna, vitamins and massage) to rid my body of toxins - so far it appears to be working. I am also eating a restrictive diet and taking a large number of vitamins and supplements designed to reset my body's immune system.

6. So what are these CD34 things anyway and how do they interact with everything else we know?

In my naiveté, I believe this is the $64,000 question. If I could get to the bottom of this one and know for sure what causes the precursor cells to be improperly marked, I would have a much clearer understanding of what may help. So far, it appears there is a definite linkage between free radicals (the presence of free radicals can alter genetic coding and cause a change in protein structure), my shortage of threonine, arginine and Cystine (amino acids) and how mutated proteins may eventually result in cancer (in my case leukemia).

7. What is the difference between leukocytes and lymphocytes?

A leukocyte is any kind of White Blood Cell. A lymphocyte is a specific type of WBC in the lymphatic system (The tissues and organs (including the bone marrow, spleen, thymus and lymph nodes) that produce and store cells that fight infection and the network of vessels that carry lymph.) So - lymphocytes are part of the immune system that fight infections. (How can Hodgkin's and AA be unrelated?)

8. I don't understand the fact that if my immune system is over-reacting, why I want to "strengthen" my immune system. As Sue explains it, my immune system is out of balance and the EI strategy is designed to get it back in balance. Need to further articulate this in a way that I understand.

According to both Dr. Lancet and Dr. Rea, I need to do "balance" my immune system and so far I think the MCS and environmental approach appears to have a better and less toxic way of accomplishing this than ATG et al.

9. Define, rationalize, categorize, synthesize and understand Cytoxan, cytokines, proteins, amino acids, CD's, folic acid, interleukins, lymphocytes, leukocytes, toxins, antibodies, antigens, magnesium, calcium, hemoglobin, hematocrits, phagocytosis, neutropenia, thrombocytopenia, T Cells, B Cells, Killer T Cells, apoptosis, fibromyalgia, immune system, thymus, tonsils, adenoids, spleen, allergies as related to immune disorders, CFS (Chronic Fatigue Syndrome, MCS (Multiple Chemical Sensitivities), detoxification vs. chelation, depuration, mitosis, vitamins (B12, E, C, A), L-Lysine, Cod Liver Oil, serotonin, glycoprotein, lymphatic system vs. lymphocytes vs. lymph nodes?

This is a tall order and is in process on a daily basis. I try to document everything that I read on the website and then relate it to my particular dilemma.

10. Why do all these other diseases keep popping up and what is the relationship with AA: AIDS, HIV, Arthritis, Lupus, Hodgkin's, TTP, ITP, MDS-RA, CFS, MCS, and Diabetes.

They are all related to the immune system. If you start by getting the immune system in balance (see above) then you can begin to address the specific issue that got your immune system out of whack in the first place. I question why everyone (and especially NIH) fails to recognize the similarities and have a centralized autoimmune effort going on rather than all the fractionalized efforts. It sucks that HIV gets all the attention when you consider how most people become infected in the first place and by the way I live in fear of one of my almost 100 transfusions passing HIV or hepatitis or some other ugly disease on to me.

* * * * *

As I am writing the book, I continue to ask these and other questions, test the answers and document what appears to be working. It is probably less scientific than many would like to see, but it is my body, my illness and it works for me.

Chapter 29

The Holistic Approach

Allowing Your Body to Heal Itself

"Just the facts, ma'am, just the facts"

Sgt Joe Friday of original Dragnet TV fame

What Has Been Tried In the Past?

A short history of medicine:

I have an earache.

2000 B.C. - Here, eat this root.
1000 A.D. - That root is heathen, say this prayer.
1850 A.D. - That prayer is superstition, drink this potion.
1940 A.D. - That potion is snake oil, swallow this pill.
1985 A.D. - That pill is ineffective, take this antibiotic.
2000 A.D. - That antibiotic is artificial. Here, eat this root.

Source Unknown

A good friend and former neighbor who knew that I was struggling with alternative approaches to curing my illness sent the above clip to me.

My quest for a cure has included both conventional and alternative strategies. My Personal Wellness Plan evolved and continues to evolve based on what I have read, researched and tried. I am continually modifying it based primarily on input from my body.

I encourage you to do your own research and make your own conclusions because everybody is different. We have ball been exposed to different things in our lives and will react differently to the various approaches that follow.

* * * * *

The National Institute of Health Office of Alternative Medicine (888- 644- 6226) is funding a number of studies to confirm the efficacy of some alternative treatments. Their budget has grown from 2 million in 1992 to 100 million for 2001. According to their latest statistics one third of Americans now use alternative treatments. 83% used these in combination with conventional medicine. In certain rural populations and in Europe the statistics reach 70%. There are move visits to alternative practitioners than primary care physicians.

Holistic Medicine is defined by the Canadian Holistic Medical Association as "a system of health care which fosters a cooperative relationship among all those involved, leading towards optimal attainment of the physical, mental emotional, social and spiritual aspects of health. It emphasizes the need to look at the whole person, including analysis of physical, nutritional, environmental, emotional, social, spiritual and lifestyle values. It encompasses all stated modalities of diagnosis and treatment including drugs and surgery if no safe alternative exists. Holistic medicine focuses on education and responsibility for personal efforts to achieve balance and wellbeing."

Alternative Medicine is often used by the general public and some healthcare practitioners to refer to medical techniques which are not known or accepted by the majority "conventional" or "allopathic" medical practitioners (usually M.D.'s). Such techniques could include non-invasive, non-pharmaceutical techniques such as Medical Herbalism, Acupuncture, Homeopathy, Reiki, and many others. However, the term Alternative Medicine can also refer to any experimental drug or non-drug technique that is not currently accepted by "conventional" medical practitioners.

As non-invasive, non-pharmaceutical techniques become popular and accepted by large number of "conventional" practitioners, these techniques will no longer be considered Alternative Medicine. Alternative Medicine refers to techniques that are not currently accepted by "conventional" practitioners, but what is currently accepted is quickly changing.

Even the definition of "conventional practitioners" is quickly changing. Therefore, techniques that are now considered part of Alternative Medicine will soon be considered part of "conventional" medicine. The terms Holistic Healing and Holistic Medicine are slightly more stable than Alternative Medicine and are therefore preferable.

Complementary Medicine is often used by "conventional" medical practitioners to refer to non-invasive, non-pharmaceutical techniques used as a complement to "conventional" medical treatments such as drugs and surgery. The term implies that "conventional" medicine is used as a primary tool and the non-invasive, non-pharmaceutical techniques are used as a supplement when needed. In many cases, properly chosen non-invasive and non-pharmaceutical healing techniques plus properly chosen lifestyle changes can completely and safely heal both acute and chronic illnesses. In other cases, "conventional" medicine is only needed in emergencies or when the safer non-invasive, non-pharmaceutical methods fail. In some cases "conventional" medicine will be a major part of a Holistic Healing Plan, but in some cases it is not needed at all.

In addition to the alternative medical treatments, I have explored and will continue to explore other elements involved in the total healing process. I am starting with reading the information at the following links: http://www.holisticmed.comhttp://www.mv.com/ipusers/howell/ejh/and has already attempted some of the yoga techniques and positions. I have a ways to go but I already know that I am recovering some of the suppleness I had many years ago. I can now fully extend to my toes and beyond both sitting and standing.

Prior to starting my holistic regimen, reaching down to touch my ankles was virtually impossible. I can now place my palms flat on the floor without bending my knees. Concentrated thinking was not possible. I would jump from subject to subject with no sense of clarity. I am now writing a book, actively trading the stock market and have the energy back from before I was sick.

By following the plan below, you can accomplish this same "revolutionary" change in less than six months. Unfortunately, one of the first steps is one of the most frightening. You have to give up the drugs that are literally killing you. As a society, we have become far too dependent on pharmaceutical cures to modern illnesses.

I do not use any medications whatsoever, use no herbal treatments and take an occasional multivitamin when I feel tired. I do take specific vitamins and minerals to replenish my system following the sauna. Otherwise, I rely completely on natural foods for the nourishment of my body.

I avoid sugar, dairy products, meats, caffeine, etc. (all the things we know are bad for us) and try to follow a rotational grains, greens and beans diet. I have dramatically reduced the stress in my life, often do conscious meditation, exercise daily, have renewed my relationship with God and have an inner peace never before experienced.

If you would like to regain control of your life, then follow the steps I describe at the end of this chapter, but first you may want to read the following:

Why should you listen to me?

I was diagnosed with Severe Aplastic Anemia in January of 2001 and was given less than six months to live. As of December 18, 2002 I am still here and about 85% of my old self. My Complete Blood Cell (CBC) counts are stable but not yet rising. My last red blood cell transfusion was on May 24, 2002 and my last platelet transfusion was on July 23, 2002.

As Dr. Kenneth Bock states in his book The Road to Immunity, "No one therapy works all the time, just as nothing is 100 percent preventive. When my patients start out with an attitude of 'This is it', I counsel them that healing is the result of hard work at many levels, and their healing regimen may involve many different treatments and approaches used simultaneously."

I have devoured books and online information regarding the various approaches to dealing with AA and other autoimmune disorders. I have read all of Dr. Sherry Rogers's books where she advises the importance of the "grains, greens and beans" diet and discusses food groups to avoid including the "deadly night shades" (potatoes, tomatoes and peppers).

She and others highly recommend the use of vitamins and supplements. Dr. Rea had me on so many supplements I felt as though I had simply swapped meds for vitamins. Dr. Rea espouses a "rotation diet" in which you can virtually eat just about anything but only every four days. He does stress that organically grown foods and free-range meats are critical in order to avoid exposure to pesticides and other chemicals.

Dr. Weill advises us to eat less protein because "residues of protein metabolism can irritate the immune system, especially in people prone to allergy and autoimmunity."

He joins other in recommending, "A low-protein, high-carbohydrate diet with plenty of fruits, vegetables, and fiber", saying that it "is good for immunity as well as general health."

He cautions: "Do not eat many foods of animal origin. Meat, poultry, and dairy products often carry residues of antibiotics and steroid hormones that can weaken immunity. Minimize consumption of milk and milk products, especially if you are prone to allergy or autoimmunity. Milk protein is a common irritant of the immune system. "

Contributors to the Aplastic Central website have recommended Chinese herbal treatments and teas, mushrooms, aroma therapy, popcorn, sesame seeds and oil, meditation, complete vegetarian diets, carbohydrate diets, all meat, no meat, fruits, no fruits, etc. I objectively read and try to understand every posting.

I may not always agree with the approach and in the end I decide what I will do, but I greatly appreciate the information that has been provided by so many well-intentioned people from all over the world. Friend and acquaintances have recommended everything from shark liver to home brew green concoctions. In the end, I tried to use my own best judgment to devise a program that so far has worked well for me. Since we are all different and live in different parts of the world with different needs and access to different resources I believe it is advisable to design and implement your own program. It is important to discuss your approach with your caretakers, but I would advise against following any one program without experimenting first.

What am I doing that works?

I am not a medical professional - I am a reasonably well-educated patient and have become my own human guinea pig in search of a cure for Aplastic Anemia. I am not selling anything or recommending any magic formula or cure all. The suggestions listed below are all free lifestyle changes that may help you in your battle to regain control of your immune system.

A key element is that you must take charge of your personal situation and think of your doctor and other health care professionals as your aids. Think about how much time your doctor spends with you in a given week vs. how much time you have available to help yourself.

Even the most well-intentioned doctor may see you only 1/2 hour per week and they have many other patients with dissimilar maladies that they must try to help.

Certainly recognize that you will need a doctor to handle the critical care and emergency situations and to monitor your progress. You will also need transfusions as long as your counts remain in a critical zone. But while this is happening, take the time to explore the alternatives available for taking control of your own destiny.

I personally intentionally avoided all the "quick fix" bottled cure-alls and opted for a holistic and natural approach. Over time, I have weaned myself off all medicines, drugs, supplements etc. The only supplements I am still using are to offset the nutrients drained from my body during sauna and detox treatments. Otherwise, my approach is completely natural and does not really cost me anything other than purchasing whole organically grown foods whenever possible and practical.

When the immune system is impaired which is the case for Aplastic Anemia and many other diseases, the body has difficulty removing toxic matter and absorbing the nutrients that keep us alive. Over time, toxins are absorbed and actually bind themselves to our cell structure. This completely disrupts normal bodily functions and we experience gas pain, constipation, and all sorts of other ugly things. Our system is literally clogged!

Along these same lines, Sue learned that when our immune system malfunctions, there is also a defect in the production of T cells and a defect in their ability to perform their designated functions. As a result, antibodies are under or overproduced. With Aplastic Anemia, the T cells destroy blood cells before they are allowed to mature. It therefore seems highly plausible that if we can fix my immune system, T cells will perform properly and my cells will be again be allowed to mature properly.

A recurring theme with many of the advocates of alternative medicine is the requirement to "heal the gut." I don't much care for their terminology, but the underlying theme appears to be solid. It goes something like this:

Over a period of many years, due to the ingestion of too many processed foods and sugar and fast food, etc. our digestive system begins to develop "leaks" and we have (you guessed it) a "leaky gut."

So, what should we do? "Heal the gut" by introducing wholesome foods back into our diet and eliminating all the bad stuff. Seems as though our digestive system gets clogged over time and it becomes necessary to purge the system and start fresh. It all seems perfectly logical to me now that I am a certified plumbing flusher!

It actually worked very well for me and I can tell almost immediately when I am eating something that is bad for me. My stomach makes all kinds of ugly noises, my throat and sinuses clog up and my heart works over time to try to help my digestive system absorb the "crap" I am eating.

By "it", I mean the cleansing process. I began by eliminating all junk food, processed foods and sugar based products. I ate only the by now infamous "grains, greens and bean" for several weeks. Everything was organically grown and I drank only fresh spring water.

At the same time, I began the detoxification process of daily coffee enemas and once I was in Texas, included a daily sauna and a "detox cocktail" consisting of tri salts, psyllium (a natural laxative) and the oil of the day (sesame, canola, olive, etc.) Believe it or not, I could actually feel my system cleansing itself and I would know immediately if I ate something that was not allowed.

The "gut healing" process is critical because without a clean "leak-proof" gut the nutrients we put into our bodies do not get properly absorbed. So, step one in the whole alternative approach is to "heal the gut."

The following is a cleaner description of the process that has evolved and continues to evolve as I become more attuned to the needs of my body.

The Personal Wellness Plan

The fundamental strategy I have adopted is to "Provide a Healthy Environment to Allow My Body to Heal Itself." This strategy has evolved a very long period of time and I encourage reading the entire book to gain an understanding of why and how this approach was developed.

1. Take the time to read everything at my site because it chronicles my journey and many others with all the ups and downs - http://aplasticcentral.org. Start and end with My Journey and this Holistic Approach. I tried ATG and the toxic drugs regimen; I was a candidate for Bone Marrow Transplant and decided against it. I was also very close to undergoing another toxic strategy using a drug called Cytoxan. I decided against all of them and have taken a "Natural or Alternative Approach". The good news is that it is not expensive - the bad news is you have to make radical changes in your lifestyle and diet and it took almost 6 months before I stabilized. I am now transfusion independent and have 85 % of my old life back!

2. Read the books by Dr. Sherry Rogers that can be found at either http://amazon.com or http://prestigepublishing.com. If possible, start with an environmental or chemical allergy doctor if you can find one. If not, maybe go online and start with http://www.macrobiotics.org/default.html

And try to build from there, using other links I provide at http://aplasticcentral.org/Alternative_Medicine/alternative.htm (bottom of page). Also check this website http://www.geocities.com/marlakins/index.html - Marla uses a vegetable based diet and is very knowledgeable on how virtually everything impacts our immune system. I use a vegetable and macrobiotic combination. Other very good sources that have been recommended by Marla and others include: http://www.gerson.org, http://www.godshealthplan.com/healthtips/healthtips.html,

3. Set a goal to become transfusion and drug independent. Maintain the transfusion regimen because it is necessary to keep you alive while you fight your fight, but set goals to lengthen the time between transfusion and then meet the goals (It takes time and there will be setbacks so also be patient with yourself). As of December 14, 2002 it has been nearly seven months since my last blood transfusion and nearly four months since my last platelet transfusion.

4. Make the necessary lifestyle changes based on the belief that AA is an autoimmune disorder and we need to help our body rebalance its immune system. Avoid the "quick fix" cures with herbs and shark oil or any "other one stop shop for a cure" Many of them may help but it is the understanding of a full program that will result in success.

5. Become at peace with yourself and your illness - If you are a "Type A", become a "Type B". Dr. Bernie Siegel says that a positive attitude is perhaps the most important ingredient in combating illness and disease.

6. Give your body the rest it is asking for - Even if it means sleeping 10 hours a night - It is literally battling for your life and needs all the help you can give it. Take naps when you feel tired, but also push yourself to exercise as much as you can.

7. Get tested for toxins by the environmental or chemical allergist and take the antigens prescribed. Avoid people who smoke, use lots of perfumes, gasoline fumes, etc. After a while you will virtually smell and feel the things to avoid. Go for fresh air and sunlight. Get a good air cleaner (mine cost about $500) and use it to clean the air in your sleeping room. Keep the dusts and pollens down.

8. Find a regimen that will help eliminate harmful toxins from your system (I take a daily sauna). Clean up your personal environment. Get rid of carpets (I moved to a different house with hardwood floors). Avoid chemicals in your house and environment. Pay very careful attention to your physical environment - Clean air? (Get a good quality air filter - $500) Mine is an Austin Healthmate (Search on Austin Healthmate at http://google.com and you'll find lots of places to buy one) Avoid toxic substances (gas, cleaning fumes, etc.).

9. Exercise at least 45-60 minutes per day You will likely have to build up to this as I could barely walk when I started)

10. What you eat is critically important and we all seem to be constantly experimenting with this facet. The one clear theme is what NOT to eat, i.e. processed foods, fast foods, "enriched" flours, etc. I personally subscribe to what I call a "rotational mostly macrobiotic diet". As much as is humanly possible, I eat Grains (30-60% of each meal), Greens (25-30%) and Beans (10-15%). This diet recommended by Dr. Rogers and I have modified it to be "Grains, Greens, Beans and Veggies." Thank goodness I like soup, because I make a lot of soup using these ingredients. This means I eat lots of Healthy Brown Rice, Oats, Barley, etc. I also try to eat only organically grown fresh vegetables and many say you should not even cook the vegetables (strictly raw fruits and vegetables) and I eat beans prepared from scratch (black, red, navy and a few others). I also eat a limited amount of meat including turkey, chicken and fish. (Once in a while I have pork even though I know it is not good for me, but it is a serious weakness.) I have successfully gotten off beef. I am quite sure that everyone's situation is a bit different and you probably need to experiment with different wholesome foods to see what it is your body needs. After a while you can actually feel what is good and what is not. Obviously avoid smoking, caffeine, drugs or any kind, processed foods (especially sugar), fast foods - All the things your mother told you would be bad for you!

11. I drink only fresh spring water courtesy of my In Laws. They have a natural spring on their property and we make a weekly trip to their property and then refrigerate the water. I strenuously avoid soda, caffeine drinks, sweetened drinks, etc.

12. I also must tell you that I do a daily detoxification program using a coffee enema as prescribed by Dr. Sherry Rogers in her books "Tired or Toxic" and described elsewhere in this book. Yuk, Ugh, etc. but it works.

13. Research and read everything you can find that discusses these alternative approaches and decide what will work best for you and be willing to a make the necessary changes. Keep a journal so you can refer back to it. You will definitely feel overwhelmed and confused at times. That is one of the reasons I keep this website active and chronicle all my successes and failures. If you falter, regroup and start over.

14. Do not lose hope or become discouraged because your outlook is critical. Maintain a positive attitude - When you lose your way, come back and read the success stories and words of hope at my site.

15. Find spiritual peace - I became active in church and strengthened my faith in God after drifting away for a long time. Every one of us needs three things: Someone to love, something to do and something to hope for.

16. Do a personal fundraiser - I had a golf tournament and raised the money I needed to attend the treatment center in Dallas (EHCD) and cover expenses not covered by insurance. My wife, daughters and friends organized it and it was very successful. I had a second one primarily to let people know that their kindness worked. It was hundreds of people giving small amounts but added up to a big enough number to cover my expenses.

17. Keep up with the forum and become an active participant. Surround yourself with positive people and bombard yourself with positive thoughts.

18. Seek God's Blessing and Good Luck in Your Endeavor!

As further evidence consider the following journal entries

August 21, 2002

Yesterday, I arose at 6:30, showered and dressed and arrived at the golf course at about 7:30 AM. My partner-brother-in-law and I, shot a combined score of 72 to tie for the lead in the top flight of our member-guest tournament.

We then played an additional 9 holes and are still tied for the lead - I played 27 holes of golf in 90 degree weather and had enough energy left to go out to an anniversary celebration dinner, watch some SU football and finally fall asleep about midnight.

Can you imagine? Last year at this time, I could not even walk up six steps without grabbing a wall to steady myself. This morning I arose again at 6:00 and a ready to go at it again.

August 31, 2002 - It's Working! I am actually running upstairs and easily walking up hills. Throw out the drugs and get on the alternative bandwagon! I am finishing up a one- week trial visit with my daughter, son-in-law and grandson in North Carolina. As soon as it snows in CNY, I am heading south as I believe that fresh air and sunshine are a necessary part of my treatment protocol.

Fast forward to January of 2003

Starting on January 3 and continuing to January 21, I launched a project to add a bonus room in Fred and Melanie's attic. I sawed boards, pounded boards, assembled walls, hung sheet rock, laid out plumbing, pulled wire and did virtually everything necessary to fully construct the new room. My energy level was incredible; I experienced several cuts and bruises and was still able to continue working 8-10 hours per day for nearly three weeks! I interrupted the effort briefly to visit a doctor and have my blood counts checked. Platelets were actually higher at 24,000 than when I left Syracuse and everything else was about the same.

For the record, Dr. Kirshner has been very supportive of my efforts. He saved my life and he and his staff (especially Nurse Klinger) nurtured me back to health so that I could try this holistic approach. They have kept an open mind and that has made it much easier for me to help my body heal itself.

Chapter 30

Insights from Marla

From Her Aplastic Central Entries

Hi Bruce: Just read your latest update and again can relate very much with your conflicts. I had avoided leafy greens for some time because of the iron issue but was also torn with the knowledge that green leafy vegetables are claimed to have other beneficial attributes. The approach I took regarding choosing what to do and not to do was based on what benefit I could obtain overall. (After all, that's what conventional medicine does also.) I know that you already understand the concept of trying to get the body back into balance for optimal health and that detoxification is necessary.

However, in addition to that, I viewed all of the body as working together as a whole, so I would try to work on overall health, not just what boosts blood counts. For instance, along with the bone marrow, other parts of the body are instrumental in blood production such as the kidneys and liver. (Actually, this is what Chinese herbalists focus on with their herbs--restore the health of the liver and kidneys because they think that is the root to many cases of blood production failure.

That is also one reason they treat many blood diseases similarly with herbs because they are trying to clean and restore the health of the liver and kidneys. This was one of my conflicts with accepting any conventional medicine because "all" the conventional treatments are toxic to the liver and kidneys.)

You may know that patients with kidney problems frequently have blood problems as well. My husband had read that there are actually hormones made by the blood vessels and the kidneys that are believed to signal the bone marrow to produce blood. With that information, I endeavored to increase the health of my kidneys.

According to Dr. Norman Walker author of Fresh Vegetable and Fruit Juices, cucumbers aide the urine production that helps the body rid itself of excess uric acid. Lemon is also thought to be a good kidney and liver cleanser.

Romaine lettuce, according to Dr. Walker, has been found to contain properties that aide the function of the adrenal cortex (which is located right on top of the kidneys). Iron appears to be one of the smallest components of romaine lettuce. Other components romaine lettuce has which are more abundant are calcium, magnesium, potassium, phosphorus, Sulphur, silicon, chlorine, sodium, oxygen, hydrogen, nitrogen, distilled water, protein, carbohydrates, fats, vitamin A, C, Thiamin, Riboflavin, and Niacin.

I believe there are likely other components that are unknown in lettuce yet are there which make all those nutrients more usable by the body. Now, if you are uncomfortable taking lettuce, I definitely understand as I was also. I've had to do things as trial and error since I didn't know anyone with my condition that had already documented their results.

Since my progress was so slow, I wanted to try something else, so I started to eat and juice romaine lettuce and have found that it did not raise my iron level. Actually, it has remained the same, and I felt better. I don't know if it was a coincidence or if in fact it was the lettuce juice, but after I started juicing lettuce for a while, my hemoglobin started to hover.

I have not used Desferol for six months now. (If my ferritin doesn't start moving down more, I may try phlebotomy provided my hemoglobin levels remain good. But, that's another issue. I'm currently working on getting my B12 in range and have a suspicion that the Desferol may have removed some of my B12 stores. I haven't confirmed that thought.)

My iron is still way too high at 1700 from latest check last month, but down from 1758 from the test the month prior to that. I have been juicing four heads of romaine a day as well as eating at least one salad a day. (I have recently reduced that to one salad most days. I'm planning to update my "sample diet for a day" on my site.)

I'm trying not to be long-winded here, but it's hard for me to explain everything clearly without going back and forth and sticking in "asides." Basically, my reason for trying the lettuce was if I could get the benefits of the lettuce at the expense of taking in more iron, well, as you know iron can be removed.

It is thought to take years for damage to occur and have you known of anyone getting iron overload from lettuce? The blood transfusions are far worse. You need to give your body what it can use. (BTW, I don't use spinach.)

Regarding lentils, I didn't know they were used for blood thinning, however, I did and do have them occasionally and seem to have no problems with them as far as bleeding or petechiae. However, if protein is what you were using them for, there are other sources that you can use instead. I don't think you'd be missing a whole lot if you omitted them from your diet.

The things I have generally stayed away from are shitake mushrooms or mushrooms in general, spinach, golden seal, Echinacea, and too many beans. One thing I think affects me with blood thinning is using too much cayenne pepper. I do still use it, but I don't use a lot at once because I think it did contribute to a slight nose bleed once which is pretty uncommon for me, but quickly resolved.

I use garlic moderately for the same reason. Going back to the lentil issue, are you presoaking your grains? I have read that you should pre-soak your beans and grains such as rice and wheat to deactivate their enzyme inhibitors and increase their nutritional value. I've attached part of an article below for you regarding this.

SOAK THOSE GRAINS

Two recent studies support the health benefits of traditional grain preparation methods. Japanese scientists found that rice that has been soaked for a day before it is cooked contains more fiber, minerals and vitamins than non-soaked rice.

The soaked rice also contains triple the amount of lysine, an important amino acid, and ten times more gamma-amino butyric acid (GABA), and a nutrient that benefits the kidneys. (Neutralization of strong chelating complexes such as phytic acid explains the paradoxical increase in mineral content.)

A 22-hour soaking in warm water allows the rice to begin the germination process, during which there is a proliferation of nutrients to feed the growing plant. The soaked rice was easier to cook and tasted sweeter (Reuters 12/12/01).

In another study, three groups of rats were fed three different sorghum porridges. One group received sorghum flour, milk solids and cane sugar cooked in water. A second group received the basic porridge inoculated with germinated grain as a source of amylase.

The third group received the basic porridge inoculated with lactobacillus planta rum to generate lactic acid for 24 hours before feeding. After four weeks, the third group of rats had better growth.

All groups took in the same number of calories but fermented porridge had higher protein values (Ahrens, FASEB Abstract, 1989). These studies highlight the importance of grain fermentation in countries where protein is scarce.

Unfortunately, in Africa, where fermented porridge and beverages were an integral part of the diet, missionaries and health workers discouraged their use because they may have contained small amounts of alcohol.

They also have a short shelf life and cannot make a profit for large corporations.

Here is a quick note on juicing. The main purpose for it is to get the maximum amount of nutrients into your body quickly. By juicing, you separate the fiber from the juice so that your body doesn't have to work at digestion. (That's why you use a juicer and not a blender.)

Theoretically, your body spends much time and energy digesting food and only takes about 30% of the nutrients through digestion whereas juiced fruits and vegetables require no digestion and the body is able to use almost 90% of the nutrients.

Since no digestion is involved, it is believed that it goes quickly into your blood stream. In that respect some use juicing as medicinal treatment. Sorry to hear about your central line problems, but when I had my PICC removed and got a routine going, it went very well for me.

I made sure I knew where the veins were that the nurses seemed to be able to hit at the first poke. I have pretty good AC veins (the ones in the bends of the arms) which I reserved for the nurses that I knew weren't as good. I reserved the harder spots for the really good IV nurses. I had about 6 areas that I would rotate so that I could give each site at least three weeks to heal in between transfusions.

My sister also had me exercise my arms with those squeeze balls. (My sister is an RN too and actually started my IV's a couple of times because she couldn't stand to see it when they missed the first time. But, until I got my system going, I had my days of playing voodoo doll.) Also, I made sure I was well hydrated since that helps to plump up your veins. When I used my AC veins, I made sure I kept my arm straight as much as possible to prevent any scarring. Scarring, as Sue probably has already told you, makes veins harder to access. I had developed sensitivity to the tagaderm so they used an ace type wrap that held my IV in place. (I forget the name of the wrap, but Sue probably knows what it is.)

Lastly, if it were me I would look at your latest BMB and compare it to your previous one and decide for yourself whether you're having "minimal" improvements or not. Doctors tend to look at things differently than we do. The comment of the "proof is in the platelets" makes no sense to me.

If you end up making your own red blood and your white counts starts to look good even if your platelets are still low, that's improvement no matter what the platelets say. I would take a look at the results myself and decide. Okay, don't mean to talk your ear off again, but there's so much to consider. I've made my mistakes along the way, but I still made improvements along the way too. I'm still learning and trying to fix my oversights. Take care, and good luck!

October 27, 2002 - Healing the Gut

Based on several recommendations by Marla, I have done some reading at the Dr. Mercola site and highly recommend you spend some time there. Dr. Mercola also directed to the link below which does an excellent job of describing how the digestive system works. I don't necessarily agree with his herbal and spinal approach to healing the gut (I am still a Dr. Rogers macrobiotic diet and coffee enema fan because it is working for me), but the explanation of the process is very good.
http://www.thedoctorwithin.com/index_fr.html

Chapter 31

Managing Out Stress

From Type A to Type B

This was perhaps my biggest challenge in deciding to fight my illness full time. Even after almost dying three times, I was continuing to try to run the business and be involved in highly stressful situations. As I went back to my notes for writing the book, I found my journal continually interspersed with new and longer lists of things I needed to do for the business.

I was trying to re-invent the business at a time when the entire industry was in a shambles (the now famous dot.com bubble was bursting) while I was laying in my hospital bed. I was also trying to save our most important client by coordinating a trip to Florida for the installation of their last server in the rollout of a four-branch installation. I could barely lift my head off the pillow yet I had to get this installation done so that we could get paid and keep from losing everything.

Thankfully this customer and especially the management team were extremely patient and compassionate. They understood our predicament but they were opening a new branch and absolutely had to have a computer available to run their business. The job needed doing and, at the time, I was the only one who had the necessary expertise. I talked Mike and Melissa through the installation from my hospital bed in Rochester!

An observation that will come as no surprise to the patients who read this book and that you must develop patience! Initially I could not believe he incredible amount of time I spent waiting in doctor's offices, waiting for breakfast, waiting for lunch, waiting for someone to deliver pain medication, waiting for ... I had never been much of a clock watcher before and had always been very impatient. I guess one positive thing that has come out of the whole experience is my newly found ability to deal with all this waiting.

I spend hour and hours and hours just sitting waiting to have my blood drawn, to see a doctor or a nurse, to be admitted to Home Tonight, to learn the results of tests, to get transfusions, etc. At times it was just unbearable for a formally very active person like me.

Friday, March 12, 2002 - My life as a "ward of the state" begins - Yes, I am "on the dole" as Ed Hayes used to say. I have completed my assignment to get ARAmatic project Phase One is now officially complete, I have removed myself from all involvement with the business, I am on Social Security Disability, we completed the move to a smaller, more affordable house, we have our financial affairs in order and I have spiritual peace.

I have, with the help of Sue, Melissa, Mike and so many others, managed the stress out of my life so that I can concentrate on getting well. My number one goal right now is to stay alive long enough to meet my soon to be born first grandchild.

I also have a new dream - to live my life for others and to provide guidance in the manner that "Ma and Pa" Burghardt have to so many young people. They are among the unsung heroes who just keep doing what needs to be done. My wife Sue inherited that disposition and to date I have only been supporting her.

It is my turn to give back and I will do my best. This book and the website are my first attempts.

Chapter 32

The Support Continues

The Bruce Lande Open is Born

Early in the summer of 2001, some of our other friends learned of the serious nature of my illness. Mark and Karen Clark with urging from Marty Bumpus, Sue's golf partner arranged a golf tournament and before the dew was off the first green, The Bruce Lande Open was born!

Melissa, Sue, the Clark's, John and Nancy Knowlton, Ron and Sue Richie, Kathie and Laverne Doctor and others worked countless hours to make the event successful beyond my wildest dreams! I was hugging people I barely knew and had to go home and take a nap while the golf was being played. Over 140 golfers turned out on a beautiful sunny day to enjoy great golf at the Links at Sunset Ridge in Marcellus, NY - Stop in if you are in the area. It is a links style course with 6 par 4's, 6 par 5's and 6 par 3's. You get to use every club in your bag and several of the par 5's reachable in two.

At the 2002 event, I not only played but also almost won the tournament. What a journey - I am now preparing to become a PGA certified professional and am shooting in the low to mid 70's on a regular basis. Given my nature, the outpouring of love and caring from immediate family and friends and even extended people I barely knew is difficult for me to comprehend. I vowed to try to be more like "these people".

I often have a hard time understanding how Sue and others can be so selfless in their effort to help others. I was humbled by the incredible amount of support provided by her family, our friends and complete strangers.

I truly had not realized how blessed I was until my ship starting sinking and I was not at the wheel. I never consciously set about building this network but I guess I had been enough of a friend to enough people at one time or another in my life that when I found myself in real trouble, the response was truly overwhelming.

As I think about it, many of the relationships were nurtured by Sue who is far better at this sort of thing than I am. She kept us in contact with some old friends who came through for us while we were in Texas and maintained contact with my relatives in the Midwest after we moved away. From Jack and Liz showing up within minutes of learning of my situation to Mark and Karen hosting a golf tournament in my honor, Melissa and Mike rescuing what was left of our failing business and Kathie and Laverne being a constant source of strength, I will never forget the kindness and generosity of so many friends, relatives and complete strangers.

Chapter 33

HOACNY & Home Tonight

They Saved My Life

Three vampires walk into a bar

The first vampire says, "Give me a blood." The second vampire says, "Give me a blood." The third vampire says, "Give me a plasma." So, the bartender says, let me get this right, "Two Bloods and a Blood Light."

I owe my life and certainly my sanity to so many caring people, but the group at the Hematology and Oncology Associates of Central New York (HOACNY) and Community General Hospital's "Home Tonight" unit certainly top the list. And the Bone Marrow Transplant Unit in Rochester follows them very closely. For nearly two years, I was completely dependent on other people's blood products to keep me alive and I became a regular at the Home Tonight, One Day Surgery department of our local hospital.

I ultimately have opted for an alternative approach to curing my illness, but I would not be here to try this approach were it not for all these caring people.

For the health care workers who may be reading this, I humbly suggest that your attitude towards your patient can be the most critical skill you possess. What may be routine to you as a caretaker, is new and frightening to your patient.

Certainly your competence is important because I had several caretakers who were obviously in the wrong profession, but what can really make the difference to a patient is the manner in which you answer questions, take the time to research concerns and generally conduct yourself around the patient and their loved ones.

The ladies in Home Tonight always went out of their way to make me feel comfortable and important and when I had not visited them in several months, one called and said:

"Hi Bruce, its Diane from Home Tonight? How are you doing? We haven't seen you in so long and we decided to check up on you."

Now, that is caring!

The manner in which the three groups mentioned above cared for me was truly extraordinary. Their warm and caring manner lifted my spirits on many days that I was about ready to give it up. I would often start my day by going to see my second favorite nurse of all time (next to Sue of course), Nurse Klinger.

Nurse Klinger is actually a Nurse Practitioner in Jeff the Elder's office and has been my primary lifeline throughout the ordeal. She has listened to all of my wild and crazy ideas and patiently brought me back to reality each time. "No matter what you do, you need to have the blood transfusions until your counts stabilize," is the most concise paraphrase of our almost weekly conversation for over two years.

Dr. Kirshner's practice, the Hematology and Oncology Associates of Central New York or HOACNY, has a stated mission of "Treating Each Life with Compassion" and I can personally attest that every single member of the staff does just that. From the receptionist who greets me at the front door to the parking lot attendant who sends me on my way at the end, every single member of the team treats me like I was the only sick person in the world.

I now have a two-year running conversation with the phlebotomy team (the people who draw my blood). I know about their kids and they ask me about mine while they are poking me with little needles and extracting my precious but limited supply of life sustaining fluid. After the blood is drawn it gets "counted" by several mysterious little machines and (when the counts are abnormally low which is always the case for me) manually confirmed. The machines actually feed blood cells through one at a time and differentiate one type from another.

While the counting is being done, I am ushered into a comfortable little room by a pleasant and efficient nurse who takes my "vitals" (blood pressure, pulse and temperature.) She runs through a checklist of questions about any abnormal bleeding, bruising, headaches, nausea, vomiting, etc., etc. I know the questions and answers by heart now and just play back my answers from a hidden tape recorder.

She smiles, I smile and I wait for either Jeff the Elder or Nurse Klinger to appear with my "counts". They show up and confirm that, yes, they are below normal and we will schedule you for a visit to Community. Most of the time, my platelet counts were under 10,000 and the concern is that anything under 10,000 could result in another "bleed to the brain" episode. I received platelets every week for well over a year.

Most weeks, virtually all of my counts were abnormal, but the ones that really matter in my case were platelets, white blood cells and hematocrits or "Crits" as we in the know tend to call them. My safe crit level is about 25 and most times they are at 22- 23 or lower so every two weeks, I would be sent for "packed red blood cells" - as opposed to unpacked I guess?

I actually tracked these counts for almost two years in the vain hope that someday they would rise rather than fall in a monotonously routine fashion. Platelets transfused into my body from others only last about six days and red blood cells last 12-14 days depending on when they were drawn from my live saving donor friends. Knowing this, I could have saved my charting effort for something more useful. The spreadsheet graph was as predictable as tomorrow's sunrise.

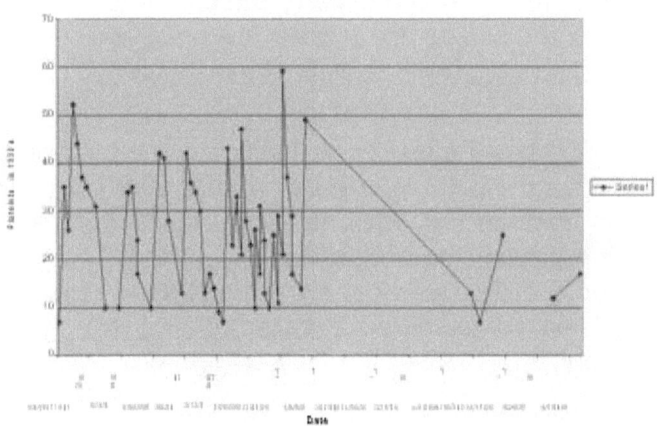

At one week, the platelet chart would drop and at two weeks, the hematocrits would drop and off I would go for another transfusion.

Upon arriving at the Community General Hospital Diagnostic Center, I would be greeted by Judy, the very friendly receptionist who would have already "fast tracked" me through the registration process since I was a regular. Earlier on, the process was not so smooth and it was very difficult for me to sit and wait being the ex-Air Force person that I am. "Go stand in that line so you are ready to stand in the next." There were even a few times that I accepted the wheel chair ride down the short hall from reception to Home Tonight.

When your blood counts are low, fatigue is the most direct effect. The red blood cells carry oxygen from your heart to the rest of your body and if there are a reduced number of these cells, your heart has to work extra hard to distribute the oxygen and carry the carbon dioxide back. When the counts are at their lowest, it is a major effort to stand up, let alone walk any distance.

My next stop in the weekly proceedings is the beloved "Home Tonight" Center where I am greeted by Diane or one of her compatriots. They have been expecting me and have my room (or in later weeks, my special transfusion cubicle), ready and waiting. Often times, the IV pump is set to go and we get started almost immediately.

For the first year of my experience, I had a "Central Line Catheter" which helped make the weekly transfusion regimen somewhat bearable, but also almost cost me my life (see the chapter on catheters and other useful devices). The attending nurse would "flush my ports" (sounds like something you do to a toilet), and give me my pre meds. The pre meds were designed to avoid allergic reactions to the foreign blood products about to be introduced into my body. I had several frightening experiences with this phenomenon before we settled on a pre-med regimen that worked.

It would start with an innocent little itch and then my whole body would swell up like a porcupine showing its needles. My whole body would be on fire from hives and I would need an epinephrine to calm me down. The magic potion for me was two Tylenol, a Benadryl capsule and a shot of hydrocortisone delivered at least 20 minutes prior to starting the transfusion.

Near the end of my transfusion experience I had opted out of the catheter game and needed and would need an Intravenous (IV) needle inserted into my arm. My veins have pretty well collapsed by this time so finding a good place to insert the needle was always a challenge. I was amazed at how well some of the nurses did this and how badly others did. It is an art form of its own and the good ones make it look easy.

So with my IV set to go, we order the blood or platelets and sit back to enjoy the day. The process usually takes a minimum of two hours from start to finish and on days when I get both blood and platelets, I can expect to spend the entire day. There were many times that I would have to start out in the Home Tonight Unit and then be transferred "upstairs" to a real hospital room for completion. This even resulted in a couple of overnight stays if I started late in the day for one reason or another.

Looking back now, the experience has made me a more patient person (pardon the pun). Prior to my illness, I was unable to sit quietly for more than five minutes. I had to be constantly doing something or planning the next thing to do. After sitting by myself for countless hours, I have learned to calm myself and appreciate the simplicity of just being alive!

Chapter 34

AA, Autoimmune and Cancer

Common Themes

I had long talks with myself about whether or not to broaden the book in an attempt to attract more readers. I ultimately chose to broaden because I believe that a major portion of the book has potential benefits for nearly everyone.

If you have one of the autoimmune related disorders then it definitely fits since it is the immune system that is malfunctioning for us AA/MDS types. If you have almost any form of cancer, it applies because the alternative remedies discussed can treat most of the cancers. This fact has been proven time and again by Dr. Rea, Dr. Rogers, Dr. Weill, Dr. Mercola, the Gerson Institute and scores of others.

If you do not have cancer, the odds are very high that someday you will unless you change the way you treat your body. I now know this to be a fact because for over thirty of my fifty years I abused my body in every way you can imagine. I smoked until my middle thirties. I was a heavy drinker until my late thirties. I ignored the signs of immune disorder such as sinusitis, tonsillitis and others. I paid little attention to the warnings on herbicides labels, varnishes, etc. and inhaled all kinds of nasty things. I was a junk food junkie. I often ate three meals a day at one food restaurant or another. I was a workaholic often putting in 16-18 hour days. I ultimately almost killed myself and my true hope is that by reading this book you will avoid many of my mistakes and take the steps now to prevent cancer from ever entering your life.

The messages in this book and the Personal Wellness Plan apply to everyone.

* * * * *

Since Aplastic Anemia and MDS are such rare diseases, there is very little written specifically about these illnesses. There is a fair amount of information on other autoimmune related disorders and volumes accumulated about cancer and specifically about alternative treatments for cancer.

The common themes seemed relatively clear and are very similar to what is working for me. Again, I personally avoided most of the concocted recipes and prefer to find my solutions naturally.

Common Themes & My Two Cents

1. Special Diets - Absolutely
2. Vitamins and Supplements - Ditto
3. Exercise - Yep
4. Free Radicals - Maybe
5. Anti-oxidants - Maybe
6. Magic Potions – Not my choice
7. Green Drinks - Nope
8. Detoxing – Need you ask?
9. Spiritual Peace – Bingo!
10. Magic Pills – Not my choice
11. Environmental Toxins – See #8

Alternative Therapy and Cancer Information

There are many other books and website that contain far more information than I could possibly report here and I encourage you to check the bibliography, the website appendix and the special resource listing at the end of this chapter.

From Ralph Moss of The Moss Reports, reportedly the World's Leading Cancer Treatment Information and Referral Service:

"It is within your reach to make the smartest possible cancer treatment decisions and give yourself every advantage in beating cancer. Let me help you discover the most advanced ideas, insider knowledge and tips, and the facts you need to wage a more successful battle. Studies have shown that doctors spend an average of 1.3 minutes answering their patients' questions. If you think there has to be a better way to evaluate your options, you are right!

I have known dozens of cancer survivors over the years and they all are independent thinkers who "color outside the lines" so to speak. Isn't that interesting? Their doctors sometimes call them "problem patients", but that doesn't deter them. They research their options and seek guidance in putting together a winning battle plan. And in many cases, these people avoid pain and disfigurement, improve their quality of life, build up their bodies and their immune system, and are alive long after their doctors said they could possibly survive. So it is not just anger that fuels me. It is also the hopeful stories of these people that keep me committed and inspired."

Alternative therapies listed on http://boobboutique.com:

Alpha-Interferon (Interferon) Hydrazine Sulfate

Anti-oxidants IP-6 (inositol, phytic acid)

Green Tea
Noni Juice
Laetrile (amygdalin)(B-17)

Anti-neoplastic Melatonin and Interleukin-2 (IL-2)
Cat's Claw (Una de gato) Mushrooms
Carnivora Pau d'Arco

Exercise Photodynamic Therapy (PDT)
Fu Zhen Potassium/Sodium
Haelan 851 Prayer

HANSI Selenium
Herbal Formulas:
Hoxey's Brew

Flor-Essence
Essiac Tea

Essiak
Canaid
ACBA

MycoStat
Shark Cartilage/Bovine Cartilage
Shark Liver Oil

Soy Products
Ukrain

Cancer Prevention

A compilation from multiple sources:

Maintain a healthy gut

Eat natural and organic fruits and vegetables
Avoid meats – use for flavoring only
Avoid processed foods of all kinds

Lose the soda, coffee and tea
Exercise at least 30 minutes every day
Drink eight 8 oz. glasses of pure water per day

Detoxify. Cleanse the body and avoid poisons.
Seek inner peace

Minimize stress when possible

Lose the booze and cigarettes
Avoid X-Rays

Cut down on the cholesterol
Strengthen the immune system
Give your body the rest it deserves

Some that I would add on my own

Stay out of hospitals

Do not accept chemotherapy
Try the macrobiotic grains, greens & beans

Pay attention to the body signals – don't mask them
Get at least 30 minutes of sunshine each day
Learn to play a musical instrument and sing

Some of the Pioneers of Alternative Cancer Treatment
(As listed on boobboutique.com)

Josef Issels*

Harry Hoxey
Max Gerson*

Linus Pauling*
Douglas Brodie
Lawrence Burton

William Donald Kelley
Isacador Emanuel Revici
Moerman

Denis Burkett M.D.
Goldberg

*See Chapter on Nutritional Healing History

Cancer and Autoimmune Related Resources

http://www.cancer.org

http://www.cancerdecisions.com

http://www.cancerdecisions.com/beatcancer_frm.html

http://boobboutique.com/aboutbreastcancer/alternatives/alternative.html

Chapter 35

Turning the Corner

Three Steps Forward

July 20, 2002 Success is at Hand

It has now been over twelve months since I decided to forego the cyclophosphamide and battle Aplastic Anemia on my terms. With encouragement and guidance from my wife, I am now becoming a true believer in the power of alternative therapies.

I am still pretty much on the rotational macrobiotic diet, take multivitamins, magnesium, and cod liver oil and essential oils on a daily basis. I was taking a lot more supplements but have dropped back to just the few mentioned previously.

I also give myself daily antigen shots and the Alpha Lymphatic Factor as prescribed by Dr. Rea. I do the sauna at least 4-5 times per week and also a bowel cleansing routine with, of all things, coffee as recommended by Sherry Rogers. I am not about to knock something that appears to be working.

I am truly feeling better every day and my time between transfusions is increasing on a regular basis (It has now been two months since my last PRBC transfusion and three weeks since I last needed platelets).

I am stronger, have virtually no limitations and have a much better outlook on the whole situation

July 28, 2002 - That Tired Old Feeling Returns

I have been extremely tired the past few days. Have been sleeping much more than normal again. It must be time for a refill - But hey it has been over two months since my last transfusion. See the doc on Thursday so will know for sure. My hematocrit was about 28 last time and holding at that level for a long time. I have been following the program pretty well so am a little disappointed but when I signed on for this gig, they told me not to be in a hurry. I am almost a year into the program and see progress but now want to put AA behind get and me on with my life.

August 1, 2002

Dr. K. says it is all right to get excited!

Jeff the Elder says that it is excellent news that I have gone 70 days since needing blood and my hematocrits are holding at 28. I wasn't sure and was pretty tired on the golf course the other day. He says it was probably the heat and that I need to be more careful than others when playing in the heat. Although 28 is good for me it is still well below normal (40-60).

But the bottom line is that I am indeed making progress with the alternative strategy and he says just keep doing what you are doing because it appears to be working!

The Red Blood Cells in my body are now my own rather than someone else's. He says that I could live many years like this! Glory Hallelujah and Thank the Lord!

August 3, 2002 Bubba and the Steep Hill

About three months ago, I went for a walk on our new street and strolled down to the bottom of our hill only to discover that I could not make it back up the hill. I had to rest about five times on the way back. Well, yesterday, I went down almost to the bottom and walked back up in one trip! This was after I had already walked 1/2 hour in the morning and about 20 minutes in the afternoon. I decided to give it a try and was amazed to discover that I am actually getting stronger.

August 16, 2002 - Let Me Count the Days

It is a little hard to believe, but it is has now been 84 days since my last Red Blood Cell Transfusion and 24 days since my last Platelet Transfusion. I continue to feel stronger every day and my count last Wednesday actually went up for the first time ever! It is a small step, but at this point a small step feels pretty darn good.

Platelets went from 12 to 14 and Hematocrits from 27 to 29 previous week. They first stabilized and now appear to actually be edging up. I am becoming even more diligent on my diet as I am swearing off red meat entirely, having a little chicken once in a while but only as a diversion rather than a major event. I am actually trying to get off that too.

I eat loads of fresh and cooked veggies, lots of lettuce, beans nearly every day and lots of rice. I can actually taste the veggies and can eat lettuce without any dressing whatsoever. In the "remember to mention department" - I use only deodorant, no antiperspirant as it keeps the toxins in one's body.

I am diligent about daily sauna and other treatments as described earlier and now take the vitamins and supplements throughout the day rather than all at the same. This allows for better absorption. Still have occasional cramping and continue to tweak the magnesium etc. to minimize this problem. All in all, the mood around here is very positive and I am beginning to feel almost normal.

August 18, 2002 - AA Patients = Super Humans

When I was the proud owner of a Hickman Catheter, I would tell my younger friends that I was an alien and that the "wires" hanging out of my chest were plugged in each night to be re-charged.

Now I have a new theory. Those of us who have AA or similar diseases are actually "super human" because our blood cells work so much better than mere earthlings. I cut myself pretty badly yesterday and my measly 14,000 platelets rushed to the scene of the accident and performed very well - let me see one of you normal types do that! Playing golf in the high 70's and expect to be breaking par before too long. - How sweet it is!

August 31, 2002 - Another Month and Battle Scars Discussion

If you have read this far, you know that I have formed a very strong opinion about the use of drugs, BMT's and other radical treatments for AA. Granted the ATG and Cyclosporine regimen did not work for me so I am certainly slated. Maybe if something had worked I would not be singing this particular tune. But alas, they did not and I reluctantly chose the "alternative approach" as a last ditch effort.

In retrospect, I see that the drug strategy, the ATG etc. are experimental efforts to combat a disease that the medical community knows very little about. When they know little about something, they do their best by throwing one experimental drug after another at it. What's worse, I was subjected to catheters, PICC lines and other stuff that almost killed me 3 times.

It was not AA that was going to kill me; it was the negative reactions to the invasions into my body. The catheter and PICC line both became infected causing sepsis (blood infection) and the ATG wiped out my immune system leaving me defenseless to even the slightest bacteria.

I now wear physical scars from the catheters and mental scars from the drug treatments. I have decided that I will NEVER again subject myself to these drugs, a BMT or any other radical treatment. I will fight AA on my terms, using my strategy and truly believe that I have a much better chance of winning the battle using this approach than any drug treatment may offer. If you have AA or some other debilitating illness or know someone who does, I encourage you to consider the lifestyle change and protocol I have described.

As for me, I am regularly playing 18 holes of golf 2-3 times per week, walking up hills, running upstairs and enjoying the company of my new grandson and other family members.

If I had stayed with the drug treatments of gone for BMT I would either be dead or have a very poor quality of life. Knowing that so many others have blindly accepted the marvels of modern medicine only to be left crippled, scarred and dead angers me.

I realize that drugs can sometimes be a good thing and that transplants are often a last resort, but I wish that doctors in general would rely less on drugs and more on insisting that we adapt the necessary lifestyle changes. Time to get off my soapbox and enjoy another day.

September 8, 2002 - Success Continues

Editorial comment: I am reporting my success as an inspiration to others. I am not boasting or "rubbing it in". I merely want those of you are losing hope to realize that we can beat this illness and at least for now, I am living proof

So.... Yesterday, I arose at 6:30, showered and dressed and arrived at the golf course at about 7:30 AM. My partner- brother-in-law and I, shot at combined score of 72 to tie for the lead in the top flight of our member-guest tournament. We then played an additional 9 holes and are still tied for the lead - I played 27 holes of golf in 90 degree weather and had enough energy left to go out to an anniversary celebration dinner, watch some SU football and finally fall asleep about midnight. Can you imagine? Last year at this time, I could not even walk up six steps without grabbing a wall to steady myself. This morning I arose again at 6:00 and a ready to go at it again.

September 19, 2002 - Counts Stable but Not Going Up

Update on the golf - we came in 5th - just out of the money but I played the full 54 holes. My next challenge is to take the PGA qualifying test on October 10th and then who knows, the title of the book could be "From AA to the PGA!" My counts today were 27 Hematocrits and 14 Platelets. I feel somewhat tired and wish they would start working their way up instead of just sitting there. Oh well, patience is definitely a virtue in this battle. I started working 8 hours a week in the pro shop to see how I handle it. So far, I am pretty tired after only a 4-hour shift! I am also back on the Desferol after a brief respite. The ferritin level is down to 800 but they want to see 500 I guess.

October 4, 2002 - A Day in My Life Now vs. Last Year - The Proof is in the "Putting"

Wow, what a difference a year makes. Yesterday I arose at 5:30, did my 45 minutes of walking and exercise, took my sauna and other treatments and was on the golf course about 8:00 (in the rain I might add), played about 14 holes bouncing around to avoid all the (other) idiots playing in the rain.

Stopped in at the clubhouse to replace a dead computer monitor for them and then headed home for lunch of navy bean soup and on to my doctor's appointment primarily just to have my CBC. Platelets were holding steady at 13.3 and hematocrits are steady at 26.6.

Returned to the golf course for another 18+ holes and figure I must have done at least 36 holes. Hit a bucket of balls to lock in the good swing feeling and headed home to get ready for Poker. Went by the grocery store to pick up snacks and a supply of grains, greens and beans. Played poker until 11:00 and fell asleep around 12:00.

That's about an 18-hour day and I was awake again this morning at 8:00. The day before (Wednesday) Sue and I went out to dinner and a movie with our good friends. For your edification, here is October 3 of last year when a trip to the grocery store was a major event:

October 19, 2002 - Counts Remain Stable & I am officially "Unusual"

	1/9/00	10/18/02
White Cells	3.5	1.6
Hemoglobin	7.3	9.7
Hematocrit	19.8	27.7
Platelets	7	15

Counts have now been stable since May 23 for RBC and Aug 23 for Platelets. Compared to original diagnosis date. They are not going up much, but they are not going down either. Whatever is there is mine.

In discussing my iron situation and whether or not to continue Desferol, Jeff the Elder says and I quote: "You are presenting an unusual case. We do not have a lot of experience with patients like you. By now, they either don't make it or they have been 'cured'".

We'll see if we can get the ferritin level down to about 500 and then you can stop the Desferol." Yippee skippee!! Oh, and BTW, I played 36 holes of golf in the PAT on October 11 and still had the energy to drive home and stay awake until normal time.

Then last Thursday; I did a full hour walk including 1/2 hour outside with "the hill" and five trips up and down stairs. I vividly remember when a slow walk up 7 steps almost did me in and a five -minute walk was an accomplishment. Made a trip to the natural food store - $50 in a mini- basket - new record for me. Also made a trip to the Onondaga Public Library and strolled the 6xx aisle for about 1--15 books which will add to my research.

November 17, 2002 - Just Catching Up a Bit

I didn't realize it, but it has been almost a month since I updated this journal. I guess I truly am returning to normal, but should report a few things. It is getting to be winter in Central New York and I can definitely smell and feel the effects of Forced Air, Natural Gas Heating. I smell it every time the furnace kicks on and wake up in the morning with that old phlegm in my throat. Yuk! Good ammunition for my going south for the winter. I am staying pretty close to my modified grains; greens and beans diet and do most of the cooking now. Because most things are from scratch it takes a good part of my time, but it fills the gaps when the market is flat.

Over the past couple of days I cleaned out my sauna room (it was packed with junk left over from the move), cleaned the laundry room, did the laundry, and made about 50 trips up and down the stairs and a ladder to the garage attic. After about 3 hours of non-stop work, had to rest for a bit. I let my heart catch up a bit and went right back to work and even had enough energy left to rake some leaves. WOW! What a difference! My counts are still lower than a normal person, but most of the time I feel pretty much normal these days.

I am still following my daily regimen which takes nearly 3 hours from start to finish, but it is well worth the effort and I look forward to the day when I can report that my counts are up to those of a normal person and I am back!

P.S. I really could live like this forever, but have this nagging concern about the counts and what might

happen if...

November 30, 2002 Journal Note

Within the past few weeks, I have received notes from the Forayer Islands (45,000 inhabitants on a small island chain between Iceland and Norway), Philippines, Australia, and many other locations. It is great to hear from all of you. Though the reason for contacting us may be sad, the support system is growing every day. My hope is that someday we will all be cured and AA-MDS and Auto Immune Diseases will go the way of Polio!

December 18, 2002 Website Update

One of the pledges I made early on is that I would always share both the ups and downs. Except for the normal battles with the IRS (which we all face), etc., I have only been reporting the upside. Well, like the song says, "Some Days are Diamonds. Some Days are Stones." I am struggling a bit of late and trying to figure out where to go from here. The most important thing I have going for me is the "someone to love" of family and friends, but there is definitely something missing. I can't seem to find the "something to do" and "something to hope for" part of the triad of happiness.

I just talked to Sue and as always; she even found a positive spin for my latest dilemma. I am frustrated by the fact that I am "on the dole" with my disability, and can't seem to find a way out. She says that's good news similar to getting cranky when you are ready to leave the hospital. I have been nosing around for job opportunities but know that I could never handle the stress of my old lifestyle. I get very uptight even thinking about it. So now my question is: "What to do with the rest of my life?" Again, from a positive point of view, there was a time not long ago, when I didn't expect to even be here!

But, let's get back on the subject. I am very depressed most days and am beginning to resent my daily routine. Less than five years ago, I had a management position with a good company, we had a nice retirement nest egg, lived in a nice house, had lots of friends and things to do and I was earning more than enough to satisfy our needs. Today, our nest egg has all but disappeared, I earn nothing and I sit here talking to myself most of the day. What makes me feel the worst is that for the first time in my life, I am unable to see a path out of the wilderness. This journal itself is just a glorified way of me talking to myself!

Yes, I know I should be happy with what I have and that I am even alive, but I am not! I have had all the free time I can handle and need to figure out a way to get on with my life. I used to dream of having this much free time to do whatever it is that I wanted to do. Now I resent it and have to figure out where to go from here.

December 20, 2002

Happy Anniversary to us! Thirty-three years ago I pledged to love, honor and obey 'til death do us part. Little did I expect that death would come knocking so abruptly.

Now there was again a light at the end of my tunnel that was not a train and I actually began to think seriously about what to do with my life again.

Chapter 36

In Search Of …

Where Do We Go From Here

Two years after I was diagnosed I stopped wondering if I would wake up the next day and stopped being paranoid about being around people. At some point in the process I realized that I was almost afraid to get better. I became paranoid about the strangest things and even when my counts finally stabilized it took a long while for me to believe it.

Once I did cross this bridge and accept the fact that I indeed may actually outlive this awful thing called Aplastic Anemia I set off on a new journey. I now needed to know what to do with the rest of my life. It was quite apparent that I would never be able to handle the stress associated with starting and running a business and my network from my days of earning over $100,000 per year at Digital was gone.

I was receiving $1700 per month from Social Security Disability, but this was hardly enough to live on and I honestly did not much care for the feeling of being "on the dole."

So the question became what to do with the rest of my life now that it looked like I would actually have one.

After kicking around Syracuse and the new small house for several months, I finally decided to head south (2 feet of snow and a temperature of –20 degrees wind chill hastened the decision) and try to sort things out a bit. I dutifully lined up a doctor in Raleigh where I would be spending the most time and checked in with Nurse Klinger prior to my departure. She assured me that I was up to the trip and wished me well.

First stop on the new life was Raleigh, NC to spend holidays with Melanie, Fred and Josh. We had a nice holiday and Sue and Melissa returned to Syracuse. I was left to play with Josh and begin a project adding a bonus room in the attic. I was hesitant at first, but then attacked the project with gusto.

I even amazed myself at what I was able to accomplish. It was like the Bubba of old. I designed, framed, sawed, pounded nails, hung sheet rock, and did both electrical and plumbing work. Fred was more tired at the end of the day than I was. There definitely appeared to be some hope that I could someday return to a normal life.

After a few brief detours in other parts of Florida to vista Michelle and Richard and some friends, I ended up in Panama City Beach on the North Gulf Coast of Florida. It is a beautiful place. I rented a place for a week and set about trying to get my new life in order.

I considered many options and still am not sure what to do. It is good to have the energy and the opportunity to even think about a life after the Aplastic Anemia experience. I had all but given up on returning to a productive life, but here I am planning for the future!

Prologue - Back to the Basics
Scrabble and Conversation

"All my life's a circle, sunrise and sundown The moon rolls through the nighttime

Till the daybreak comes around

All my life's a circle, I can't tell you why The seasons spinning round again

The years keep rolling by."

Harry Chapin

Today is Sunday, December 1, 2002. Sue slept late so I decided to put the finishing touches on the first draft of the book. I was having difficulty getting all my notes and resources organized and it finally just all came together and I have now been typing, cutting and pasting almost nonstop since eight o'clock this morning. The book will be finished shortly and then it will be on to finding someone who will publish it.

I stopped long enough to have my breakfast of oatmeal and my lunch of boiled vegetables accompanied by scrabble and conversation. Sue and I had drifted apart over the years and I thank Aplastic Anemia for bringing us back together. Before Michelle was born, we would play scrabble and talk while I was stationed in Berlin. We were in our early twenties, thousands of miles from home and barely had enough money to feed us.

We lived in a tiny apartment "on the economy" which was a polite way of saying the military did not provide housing or even housing allowances for married enlisted men. Mother Burghardt (Sue's maiden name) would send us a twenty-dollar bill for every holiday and sometimes just because she wanted to send us a card. We told her years later that it often meant the difference between having two or three meals that day. Since we didn't have enough money to do much else and had only one TV station, we passed many hours per day playing Scrabble.

We played nearly every day and learned to love each other. (We had only known each other for six months before getting married and came from two different parts of the country) I am happy to say that we are back to playing scrabble, our love is stronger than ever and I owe it all to Aplastic Anemia, Sue's love, the caring of our family and friends and a new found relationship with God.

Again I say to the IRS, "When I am dead, will you come after my wife to pay the $15,000 tax bill?" Knowing them, I am quite confident they will not let this sleeping dog lie, so in addition to the pain of losing me, she will have to deal with the relentless pursuit of the tax collectors. Therefore, I cannot die. I must live on to fight the insurance company, the illness and my old friends - the IRS.

Seems like every time I was about to get ahead in my life, the IRS would show up and say - "Wait just a minute mister, you owe us taxes from 3 years ago when you forgot to report that your dog was hit by a car and you deducted the cost of the medical treatment." The original tax adjustment was $23.18 but the interest and penalty brings your total tax bill to $875. Never mind it took us three years to find it, it was your fault in the beginning so you must pay!" I may not beat them, but I'm going to die trying.

Now that I have two Christmas seasons behind me, I begin to think that I may actually succeed in my battle, yet I had the strongest feeling standing in the communion line last month. For only the second time in my life, I actually heard God's voice telling me that this would be my last Christmas and I should enjoy this bonus time he had given me. I sometimes wonder if I am now just nervous about the prospect of getting better - like is this for real or am I just kidding myself. Another part of me sometimes feels guilty about still being alive when so many others who used to frequent the website or I learned about through friends is now gone.

My fingers unconsciously trace the scar on my right chest where the Hohn catheter nearly caused my death - not from aplastic anemia itself but from the blood infection. Nobody really dies from Aplastic Anemia – they die from a complication like a blood infection or pneumonia or graft versus host disease. I hear the clock on Melanie's wall chime "Joy to the World" and wonder if I will be here for yet another bonus Christmas.

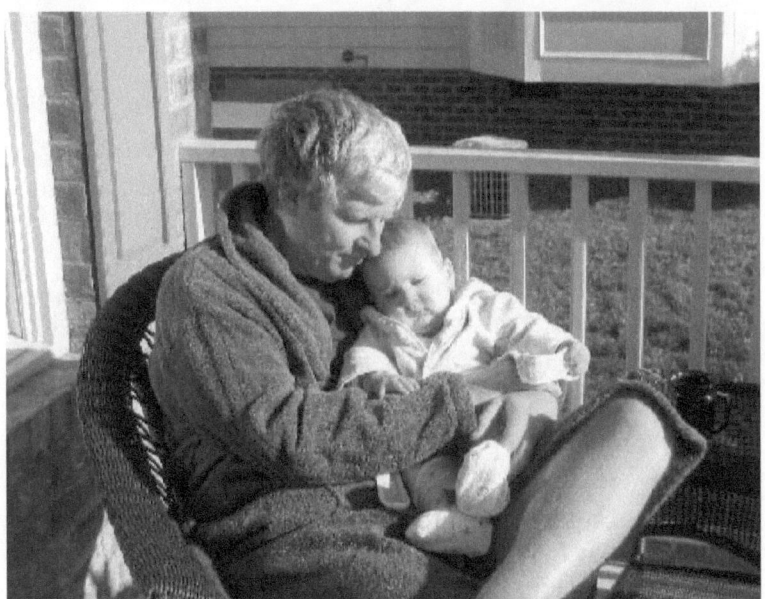

This shot was taken on Josh's nine month birthday and is the best reflection of my joy at being alive long enough to enjoy the first of what I hope will be many grandchildren and, who knows, maybe I'll even get to meet some of my great grandchildren!

I thank God every day for giving me a second chance at life and I owe it all to Aplastic Anemia, my wife Sue, my family and close friends.

Thanks!

February 4, 2003 Update

"Good Morning Mr. Phelps," as the old TV series Mission Impossible used to begin....

It is Tuesday, February 04. The temperature on the beach today is 65. As I complete the draft I am sitting on the beach in Panama City, Florida – "The Most Beautiful Beaches in the World". Back home they are suffering from one of the coldest winters in recent memory and thanks to Sue I am able to avoid the cold and finish this book.

Good News!

Sue called today and informed me that the IRS has accepted the explanation from our CPA and we no longer owe the $15,000.

I have now decided that I am officially a survivor and once the book is finished will be looking forward with what to do with the rest of my life!

As always, should you or any member of your IMF team be killed or cancelled, the secretary will disavow and knowledge of your or your team. This tape will self-destruct in 60 seconds. Good day, Mr. Phelps."

The author is not a medical professional. This book is a guide to help you understand more about your illness and present alternative methods for healing your body. Please contact your caretakers before using any of the information presented.

AA Question and Answer

What causes Aplastic Anemia?

It is for the most part considered to be idiopathic (unknown cause), but secondary AA is linked to chemotherapy and other toxic drugs. There is considerable speculation that primary AA may be caused by benzene, toxic substances in the environment, various chemicals, and the amalgams used in dentistry and many prescription drugs, but there is supposedly no conclusive evidence.

How often does it occur?

There are between 2 and 12 new cases per million population reported annually. MDS is a bit more common with approximately 50 new cases per million per year. Most MDS cases are in people over 50.

Is it hereditary?

One may inherit a "predisposition" towards the illness, but AA itself is not hereditary.

How are AA and MDS diagnosed for sure?

Through the use of a Bone Marrow Biopsy in which a small piece of bone marrow is extracted from the pelvis or other large bone and laboratory analysis is performed.

What are the laboratory characteristics of each?

Both are forms of bone marrow failure of the inability of the bone marrow to produce an adequate supply of normal healthy blood cells.

In AA, the bone marrow appears empty or is replaced by fat and there is a reduction in the normal development of healthy blood cells. Cells bearing the CD34 antigen are virtually absent in blood and marrow.

Cells capable of forming new blood cells are severely reduced.

With MDS, the bone marrow is said to be hypo cellular, meaning there is a reduced quantity of megakaryocytes (blood cell precursors). The clinical definition of Myelodysplasia is "abnormal or defective formation of the bone marrow cells."

There are also several different categories of MDS related to the presence or absence of "blast" cells, the stages of advancement towards leukemia and other factors. I have not studied MDS as closely for obvious reasons, but the AA-MDS list serve at http://aafa-ner.org/aa-mds/is frequented by many MDS patients who have a wealth of knowledge about their affliction.

So at the risk of oversimplifying these complex illnesses, with AA, the megakaryocytes are almost nonexistent and with MDS they are malformed. In both cases, the inability of the bone marrow to produce an adequate supply of blood cells is the root of the issue.

How many transfusions did you receive?

Early on I was carefully documenting everything, but at some point I stopped counting because I thought it was going to go on forever. The best I can figure, I received over 75 platelet transfusions and somewhere between 35 and 50 blood transfusions during the 17 months I was transfusion dependent.

What are the predominant symptoms?

Petechiae – Small red marks where capillaries burst
Nose and gum bleeding

Unexplained bruising
Fatigue, chest pain and shortness of breath Low Blood Cell Counts (Pancytopenia)

What is the clinical definition of AA?

This form of anemia (Too few red blood cells in the bloodstream, resulting in insufficient oxygen to tissues and organs) occurs when the bone marrow ceases to sufficient red and white blood cell production. It may be induced by exposures to high levels of toxic chemicals, radiation and certain drugs.

AA is generally unresponsive to specific therapy, often accompanied by granulocytopenia (a reduced number of white blood cells) and thrombocytopenia (a decrease in the number of platelets in the blood, resulting in the potential for increased bleeding and decreased ability for clotting), in which the bone marrow may not necessarily be hypo cellular or hypo plastic (underproduction of red blood cells) but fails to produce adequate numbers of peripheral blood elements. The term actually is all-inclusive and most probably encompasses several clinical syndromes.

What are the Standard Treatments?

1.   An option for people who are lucky enough to have an exact "HLA" matched sibling is a matched sibling (one of your brothers or sisters has the same HLA typing as you do) transplant. The odds are not the greatest, but it is the current preferred "curative" strategy.

2.   Treat the symptom and hopefully put the disease into remission using serum from a horse or a rabbit (ATG) followed by daily doses of cyclosporine which is a medication used primarily to address potential rejections by organ transplant patients. They stumbled onto the fact that cyclosporine can put AA into remission a few years ago so that is what they are using as a primary remission strategy. It works for 75% of patients, but did not work for me. Others recommend similar extremely toxic drugs including Cytoxan and MMF.

3. Undergo a Matched Unrelated Donor ("MUD") transplant. The odds for survival are very low (less than 25% of patients survive and lead anything close to a normal life).

What Alternative Treatments are Available?

Read this book, especially the chapter on holistic healing.

What is iron overload and what can be done about it?

Iron overload (hemochromatosis) occurs when an AA or MDS patient has received too many red blood cell transfusions. The body is unable to rid itself of the naturally occurring iron that has been infused from others and a ferritin test reveals abnormally high levels of ferritin in the blood.

Under normal conditions, there is approximately 4-6 gm of iron in the body. On March 1, 2002, my ferritin level was 2857 vs. a norm of 22-415 ng/ml in a male over 45 (Females over 45 s/b 15-200, females 18-45 = 6-115 and male 18-45 22-340). The body is unfortunately very efficient when it comes to storing iron

These high levels of ferritin or iron can eventually cause severe damage to the liver.

The standard procedure for removing iron is the delivery of an iron chelation drug called Desferol that has the same dangerous side effects as any prescription drug.

See http://www.ironoverload.org/ for additional information on hemochromatosis.

Medicine & Vitamin Lists

Nutrient	Benefit	Sources
Additives	Prevent spoilage & rancidity, enhance flavor & appearance, boost nutritional content	-
B Vitamins	See Individual Vitamin B's	

Nutrient	Function	Food Sources
Beta Carotene	Food containing Beta Carotene is converted to Vitamin A in the Liver.	
Biotin	Aids in cell growth and metabolism of carbs, fats and Proteins. Promotes healthy bone marrow.	Cooked egg yolk, fish, meat, milk, poultry, soybeans, and whole Grains, yeast.
Calcium	Keeps bones strong and prevents them from becoming brittle.	
Carbohydrate		
Choline	Regulation of gall bladder and liver function.	Egg yolks, legumes, meat, milk, and whole grain cereals.
Chromium	Helps maintain the body's balance of glucose (blood sugar) and is required for the body to release the energy from the glucose	
Coenzyme Q10	A vitamin-like substance that resemble Vitamin E but may be an even	Mackerel, salmon, sardines.

	more powerful antioxidant.	
Copper	Helps absorb iron and heals wounds	
Cycloallin	Anticoagulant helps protect against heart disease	
Folate	Essential for new cell development, important in DNA synthesis and cell division and replication.	Barley, beans, bran, brewer's yeast, brown rice, cheese, chicken, orange, leafy greens, lamb, lentils, pork, root vegetables, salmon, tuna, whole grains, yeast
Histidine	Needed for growth and for the repair of tissue, as well as the maintenance of the myelin sheaths that act as protector for nerve cells. It is further required for the manufacture of both red and white blood cells, and helps to protect the body from damage.	
Iron	Essential for the	

	transport and release of oxygen throughout the body
Isoleucine	Promote muscle recovery after physical exercise and on its own it is needed for the formation of hemoglobin as well as assisting with regulation of blood sugar levels as well as energy levels. It is also involved in blood-clot formation.
Leucine	Leucine helps with the regulation of blood-sugar levels, the growth and repair of muscle tissue (such as bones, skin and muscles), growth hormone production, wound healing as well as energy regulation. It can assists to prevent the breakdown of muscle pro

Lysine	It is required for growth and bone development in children, assists in calcium absorption and maintaining the correct nitrogen balance in the body and maintaining lean body mass. Furthermore it is needed to produce antibodies, hormones, enzymes, collagen
Magnesium	Helps maintain healthy energy production processes, bones, muscles and nerves.
Protein	Essential Building Block of Life
Selenium	Supports Vitamin E May be useful in preventing cancer
Threonine	It is required to help maintain the proper protein balance in the body, as well as

assist in the formation of collagen and Elastin. It is further involved in liver functioning (including fighting fatty liver), lipotropic functions when combined with as

Tryptophan — Required for the production of niacin (vitamin b3). The human body to produce serotonin, a neurotransmitter that is important for normal nerve and brain function, uses it. Serotonin is important in sleep, stabilizing emotional moods, pain control, in

Valine Needed for muscle metabolism, repair and growth of tissue and maintaining the nitrogen balance

Vanadium

Vitamin	Benefits	Sources
Vitamin A	Prevents night blindness, eye problems and skin disorders. Enhances immunity. Acts as an antioxidant and helps protect cells from disease.	Fish liver oils, animal livers, green & yellow fruits & veggies.
Vitamin B1	Enhances circulation and blood formation. Stable Appetite	Dried Beans, brown rice, egg yokes, fish, liver, peanuts, peas, pork, poultry, soybeans, grains.
Vitamin B12	Prevents anemia. Protects your nervous system and supports both bone growth and metabolism	Blue cheese, cheese, clams, eggs, herrings, kidney, liver, mackerel, milk, seafood, tofu.
Vitamin B2	Riboflavin aids your eyes and works for healthier skin and energy metabolism.	Beans, cheese, eggs, fish, meat, milk, poultry, spinach, yogurt.
Vitamin B3	Niacin helps your metabolism, improves the condition of your skin, and supports both the digestive and nervous systems	Beef, broccoli, carrots, cheese, corn flour, eggs, fish, milk, pork, potatoes, tomatoes, whole wheat

Vitamin	Function	Sources
Vitamin B5	Needed to produce vital steroids and cortisone in the adrenal gland - The anti-stress vitamin.	Beans, beef, eggs, fish, pork, vegetables, whole wheat.
Vitamin B6	Needed for DNA and RNA synthesis. Allows you to think more clearly, supports the immune system and hormone activity	Brewer's yeast, carrots, chicken, eggs, fish, meat, peas, spinach, sunflower seeds, walnuts, wheat germ
Vitamin C	Helps prevent disease and infection and promotes the body's absorption of iron. It also helps bones grow, is involved in the formation of scar tissue, and strengthens the blood vessels	
Vitamin D	Vitamin D fortifies the bones and plays supporting	

	roles in the maintenance of your brain, pancreas, skin, muscles, reproductive organs and immune system.	
Vitamin E	Helps give you healthy skin, can heal scars, and even protects the lungs from air pollutants	
Vitamin K	Needed for blood clotting and may play a role in bone formation. Converts glucose into glycogen for storage in liver.	Alfalfa, broccoli, leafy vegetables, soybeans, molasses, brussel sprouts, cauliflower, egg yolk, liver, oatmeal, oats
Zinc	Heals wounds and aids in making genetic materials and proteins.	

DEFICIENCY SYMPTOMS: May result in pellagra, gastrointestinal disturbance, nervousness, headaches, fatigue, mental depression, vague aches & pains, irritability, loss of appetite, insomnia, skin disorders, muscular weakness, indigestion, bad breath, canker sores.

CHOLINE

IMPORTANCE: Very important in controlling fat & cholesterol buildup in the body. Prevents fat from accumulating in the liver. Facilitates the movement of fats in the cells. Helps regulate the kidneys, liver & gallbladder. Important for nerve transmission and helps improve memory.

DEFICIENCY SYMPTOMS: May result in cirrhosis and fatty degeneration of the liver, hardening of the arteries, heart problems, and high blood pressure, hemorrhaging kidneys.

VITAMIN D

IMPORTANCE: Improves absorption and utilization of Calcium and Phosphorous; required for bone and teeth formation; maintains a stable nervous system and normal heart action.

DEFICIENCY SYMPTOMS: May lead to rickets, tooth decay, softening of bones, improper healing of fractures, lack of vigor, muscular weakness, and inadequate absorption of calcium, retention of phosphorous in the kidneys.

CALCIUM

IMPORTANCE: Builds and maintains bones and teeth; regulates heart rhythm; eases insomnia; helps regulate the passage of nutrients in and out of the cell walls; assists in normal blood clotting; helps maintain proper nerve and muscle function; lowers blood pressure; important to normal kidney function and in current medical research reduces the incidence of colon cancer, and reduces blood cholesterol levels.

DEFICIENCY SYMPTOMS: May result in arm and leg muscles spasms, softening of bones, back and leg cramps, brittle bones, rickets, poor growth, osteoporosis (a deterioration of the bones), tooth decay, depression.

SELENIUM

IMPORTANCE: A major antioxidant nutrient protects cell membranes and prevents free radical generation thereby decreasing the risk of cancer and disease of the heart and blood vessels. Medical surveys show that increased selenium intake decreases the risk of breast, colon, lung and prostate cancer. Selenium also preserves tissue elasticity; slows down the aging and hardening of tissues through oxidation; helps in the treatment and prevention of dandruff.

DEFICIENCY SYMPTOMS: May result in premature aging, heart disease, dandruff, and loose skin.

OMEGA 3 FATTY ACIDS (EPA & DHA): EPA & DHA are present in fish body oils and have the potential for improving the health of the cardio-vascular system. Medical reports show that as the amount of EPA in the diet increases, the risk of coronary heart disease decreases. In a nutshell, EPA from fish oils lowers serum cholesterol & triglyceride levels, make your blood less viscous, thinner & less sticky, less prone to clump together. Diets of Eskimo and coastal Japanese are rich in the Omega 3 fatty acids, EPA & DHA. Their death rate from heart attacks is much lower when compared to the Western man. DHA is a major component of the brain and retina, and has a possible role in nerve transmission. Research has shown that many migraine headache sufferers have experienced some relief from consuming Fatty Acids.

TAURINE (Non-Essential Amino Acid) helps stabilize the excitability of membranes that is very important in the control of epileptic seizures. Taurine and sulfur are considered necessary for the control of many biochemical changes that take place in the aging process; aids in the clearing of free radical wastes.

GLUTAMIC ACID (Non-Essential Amino Acid) Considered to be nature's "Brain food" by improving mental capacities; helps speed the healing of ulcers; gives a "lift" from fatigue; helps control alcoholism, schizophrenia and the craving for sugar.

HISTIDINE (Non-Essential Amino Acid) is found abundantly in hemoglobin; has been used in the treatment of rheumatoid arthritis, allergic diseases, ulcers & anemia. A deficiency can cause poor hearing.
Lab Testing Results

TRIGLICERIDES (HIGH) Mine are 216/224 vs. a norm of less than 150. A type of fat produced by your body, a mild risk factor for coronary artery disease. Best checked after a 12 hour fast. Very diet sensitive compared to cholesterol levels.

THREONINE (LOW)(Essential Amino Acid) Mine is 5.83 vs. average between 8.85 & 19.40 Is an important constituent of collagen, Elastin, and enamel protein; helps prevents fat build-up in the liver; helps the digestive and intestinal tracts function more smoothly; assists metabolism and assimilation.

ARGININE (Non-Essential Amino Acid) (LOW) 5.5 vs. Average 6.85 - 15.60 Studies have shown that is has improved immune responses to bacteria, viruses & tumor cells; promotes wound healing and regeneration of the liver; causes the release of growth hormones; considered crucial for optimal muscle growth and tissue repair. GLYCINE (Non-Essential Amino Acid) (LOW) 19.0 vs. AVG 19.8 -47 Helps trigger the release of oxygen to the energy requiring cell-making process; Important in the manufacturing of hormones responsible for a strong immune system.

GLUTAMINE (LOW) 39.1 vs. 42 - 82 is classified as a nonessential amino acid since various tissues such as the skeletal muscles, liver, and adipose tissue can readily synthesize it. However, research indicates that glutamine is conditionally essential when the metabolic demand for glutamine exceeds the amount available in the free glutamine pool and which can be provided by de novo synthesis

SERINE (Non-Essential Amino Acid) (LOW) 7.7 vs. AVG 8.5 -18 A storage source of glucose by the liver and muscles; helps strengthen the immune system by providing antibodies; synthesizes fatty acid sheath around nerve fibers.

3-METHYLHISTIDINE HIGH .66 vs. 0 - .55 an indicator of muscle damage (protein breakdown) that can be measured with urine test. Causes of elevated 3-methylhistidine include weightlifting, heart attack, etc. The ratio of 3-methylhistidine to creatine may be an important indicator for weightlifters who are trying to avoid the catabolic effect of over-training.

METHIONINE (LOW) 1.87 vs. 1.95 - 4.10 Low - possible poor- quality protein diet. May have adverse effects on sulfur metabolism. Improve dietary methionine intake or take a supplement.

FOLIC ACID they've had me on this since day one. IMPORTANCE: Necessary for DNA & RNA synthesis, which is essential for the growth and reproduction of all body cells; essential to the formation of red blood cells by its action on the bone marrow; aids in amino acid metabolism.

TYROSINE (Non-Essential Amino Acid) (LOW) 3.74 vs. 4.85 - 12.60 Transmits nerve impulses to the brain; helps overcome depression; Improves memory; increases mental alertness; promotes the healthy functioning of the thyroid, adrenal and pituitary glands.

TAURINE (Non-Essential Amino Acid) Helps stabilize the excitability of membranes which is very important in the control of epileptic seizures. Taurine and sulfur are considered to be factors necessary for the control of many biochemical changes that take place in the aging. Taurine level appears to be okay but Ron has me taking it anyways? 4.95 vs. 4.75 - 15.5

These vitamins and supplements were taken during the critical detoxification and rebuilding stages. Once I became stable, I discontinued everything except the multivitamin and the supplements necessary to replenish my body after detox treatments or sauna.

The Insurance Battle

"If the oil light on your car goes on, you can always unscrew the bulb, smash it with a hammer or buy a new car. That's analogous to the kind of medicine insurance company's pay for: drugs, drugs and more drugs." Dr. Sherry Rogers

I wrote a letter to Sue's insurance company, AKA POMCO, the "Experts in Self Insurance" on December 10, 2001 and after several stalls, they finally sent this letter in October of 2002. Is that almost a full year or have I lost touch with reality?

"Dear Ms. Lande:

This letter is in response to a request for benefit information for "allergy related services" rendered at Environment Health Services of Dallas.

Our recent review, performed by a peer medical consultant, recommended payment for multiple complete blood counts and would and blood cultures, as well as toxicology testing after confirmation that toxicology testing had not been performed. These services, the blood counts, cultures and toxicology testing, have been benefited in full (I think we have received about $1,000 vs. about $15,000 of submissions) per the terms of your Health Benefit Plan.

However the consultant noted that intradermal testing and immunotherapy are "clearly not medically necessary or appropriate for the diagnosis of aplastic anemia." The consultant noted the "discussion of the presence of seasonal allergies and chronic sinus infections affecting the patient's immune system" and concluded that the skin testing and immunotherapy done were not related to the diagnosis or treatment of aplastic anemia and is not medically necessary.

Therefore, under the terms and limitations of your Health Benefit Plan as noted in our letter of June 20, 2002, no further benefits are available for services rendered at Environmental Health Services of Dallas.

Sincerely,

Sally K. Frank, R.N.
Medical Analyst"

Now, I must admit, I feel much better knowing that an unnamed "consultant" and Ms. Frank, the world renowned expert on immunology have taken so long to carefully consider our case (A year?) and in the end, have decided that Dr. Neil Young (the real world renowned expert on AA who states: "More recently, an active role of the immune system in marrow destruction has been recognized. In 1999, most patients can be treated effectively either by replacement of the marrow through stem cell transplantation or by drugs that suppress immune system function..."), Dr. William Rea (First World Chair in Environmental Medicine) and Dr. Sherry Rogers (Author of 12+ books on how our immune systems is being destroyed by the toxins in our environment and/or the foods we eat) don't know what they are doing and we must therefore pay for all of their life-saving treatments out of our own pockets.

Dr. Rea and the preceding referral by Dr. Sherry Rogers (on the insistence of my wife, I might add) saved my life! Sue and I are the only one who really know for sure, because we have been battling this thing side by side for nearly two years. The conventional treatment was not working; it was killing me. I narrowly escaped death on four separate occasions while being administered the drugs and other treatments recommended by the conventional wisdom.

It was only after completely detoxifying my system and determining what was causing my problems in the first place that I began to turn the corner. In addition to the lifesaving efforts of Dr. Kirshner and his staff, I now have to thank Dr's Rea and Rogers for giving me back my life. I am certainly not fully recovered, but my quality of life has returned to 85-90 per cent of what it was and I have a certain level of confidence that if I get on the program and consistently stay on the program they recommend, I will ultimately beat this monster tagged "Aplastic Anemia".

When my blood counts reach a level that will provide undisputed evidence, I will again go after the insurance company and this time with a lawyer by my side. I will do it not only for my wife and me but for the countless thousands of others who have been turned down by their pharmaceutically sponsored insurance carriers. If it's not a patent protected drug, it can't work, can it? (BTW, along the way, I was prescribed and they paid for SMZ-TMP, Celebrex, Propanol, Metronidazole, Cipro, Prilosec, Lorazepam, Desferol, Diflucan, Vioxx, Cyclosporine, Prednisone, Vancomycin and a few dozen more). None of that stuff was working and in fact, it was killing me!

I now have two new goals:

1.   Become a Professional Golf Association member so I can write my book "From AA to the PGA", and

2.   Get my CBC's to a level that will provide irrefutable proof that my insurance company is wrong and get them to pay for my treatments.

Maybe I should thank POMCO, The Self Proclaimed "Experts in Self Insurance" because without them, I would not be as driven. I have always enjoyed a good fight!

Oh and, by the way, if I previously suggested that some of you go to the Patient Advocacy Foundation for help, don't bother. They are useless! After several weeks of phone tag and useless conversation they opted out on trying to help me. Thanks for nothing!

Releasing my anger and directing it at the appropriate recipients is good for the soul! I feel so much better now, and I will be sending a sanitized version to the insurance company, AKA "The Experts in Self Insurance".

Tricks of the Trade

Things we wish someone had told us...

1. If you have Aplastic Anemia or MDS, the odds are very good that you will survive, but you need to take charge of your situation and your health.

2. The drugs prescribed for treatment will make you sick. They have many potential side effects and contra-indications. Be wary of everything that you ingest!

3. The odds are high that you will have some kind of central line installed. Read the chapter on catheters, what to expect and realize that these devices offer quick access to your heart – for blood products and meds and for germs!

4. Do not swim with a central line installed

5. Do not let your site get and stay wet. The moisture provides an excellent place for bacteria to grow.

6. Do not touch or let anyone else tough your site without clean hands and gloves

7. If you are being cared for by someone who does not care or is incompetent, politely ask to see a supervisor and get a new caretaker

8. Do not assume hospitals are clean or a good place to be. They are not. The people in hospitals are sick and germs are everywhere. Do not expect to get any rest and resolve to get out as quickly as possible

9. Purchase a good quality (Austin makes several) air cleaner for your bedroom and use it. Lose the carpet in your house and especially in your bedroom. The dust and mites in carpets can be deadly.

10. If you develop iron overload from too many transfusions, opt for the sub cutaneous pump rather than having the Desferol delivered via intravenous drip.

11. As you advance with your understanding of the illnesses, it is important to go back and reread items you encountered before because with a renewed understanding you will undoubtedly discover something you missed the first time

Last Pages

A Final Message from the Author

Aplastic Anemia is an illness that can be beaten. When first diagnosed, this seemed hard to believe, but it is true. This malady and most other diseases of the 20th and 21st century are often caused by poor diet and nutrition, our environment and/or the drugs we have taken to combat the toxins to which we have been exposed.

There are many books and websites that discuss autoimmune diseases, alternative treatments, nutritional healing and holistic medicine. Why would you want to invest your time and money on yet another one?

What sets this book apart is the "no holds barred" approach to everything we tried. I abused my body for over forty years and ignored the signals my immune system was trying to send me. I literally almost killed myself before I woke up and made the necessary changes in my diet, lifestyle and environment.

Once diagnosed, my illness was approached with the same passion as everything else in my life. The result is a continually updated website containing over 200 pages and this book.

If you are willing to invest the time to understand the lessons presented in this book, you can regain control of your health and life. It will not be easy. It will require a dedicated and concentrated effort on your part but in the end you too can regain your health and restore your inner peace.

At the time of my diagnosis, I was 52 years old and in very good health for someone approaching his "golden years." We had recently expanded our computer and website business to include ten employees in two states and had moved into a larger home in the city of Syracuse.

When the doctors told us there was very little chance of a durable cure to my illness, we set out to learn everything we could, what caused it and how it could be treated. My body would be used as a human guinea pig while we tried both conventional and alternative treatments.

As is my custom, this new challenge was approached like a project complete with goals, action items, deadlines to be met and good documentation.

This book does not offer a quick fix because there are no easy answers. You won't be able to take a pill and be magically cured. Contrary to what the pharmaceutical industry wants you to think, there is no magic purple pill for everything that ails us. The pills simply mask the symptoms of what is happening to our bodies while our immune systems try to fend off the latest assault.

"I took my troubles down to Madam Ruth, You know that gypsy with the gold capped tooth. She looked at my palm and she made a magic sign, she said what you need, boy, Love Potion Number Nine"

Sue has been researching environmental medicine for nearly twenty years. Together, we developed a Personal Wellness Plan. The information presented will document what has worked for me with a very specific focus on helping my body heal itself through the use of proper diet, nutrition, exercise and attitude.

We are not recommending any miracle drugs, potions concocted from sharkskin or barley grass or other magic cures. You don't have to sign up for a newsletter or purchase a lifetime supply of anything.

Everything you need to develop your own Personal Wellness Plan is available from nature. Most of the nutrients your body needs can be found in sunlight, fresh spring water and the everyday foods you can grow yourself.

If, like me, you are not into gardening, you can buy the foods you need from a natural food store or the organic section of your local grocery store. (If you are lucky, there is a Whole Foods Market near you. If not, encourage your local grocer to add and publicize an organic section –You will both be pleased with the results.)

Refer to http://aplasticcentral.org as I update the information that can help you save your own life. As you read my story, remember there are no magic cures, your doctor is at best only a facilitator and blaming others or your situation is a complete waste of time. You ultimately must decide to take control of your life and this book can be the start you need.

Return to a natural holistic life and then share your success with others. Join the free forum or send a note to the email address on the website.

Aplastic Anemia – A Blessing or a Curse?

Thanks to my battle with Aplastic Anemia, I was able to spend an unbelievable amount of time with our new grandson Joshua. I saw him sit up, scotch, crawl, stand, walk with a walker, and investigate everything in sight. It was a marvelous experience that I would have missed had it not been for my recuperative period in North Carolina with Melanie, Fred and Josh.

I was also fortunate enough to rebuild my relationship with my wife and partner of 30+ years and get to know my children and their spouses on a new and better level. I strengthened many friendships, met a host of new friends and renewed my relationship with God.

In the end, I would honestly say that Aplastic Anemia has been a blessing and I hope that I will always look back on this time of my life with the same positive attitude.

The Readers Digest Version of My Story

I was diagnosed with Severe Aplastic Anemia in January of 2001 and given six months to live. After having my life saved by Dr. Jeff Kirshner, I entered the world of modern medicine. I was subjected to two rounds of a potent drug regimen intentionally designed to destroy my immune system, experienced life-threatening septicemia three times, consumed more drugs than I could count and almost died several times before coming to my senses.

In August of 2001, I finally listened to my wife who has been researching environmental medicine for over twenty years. Since that time, I have been following a holistic regimen that is considered an alternative to modern medical treatments but it has saved my life.

A holistic approach to life is working for many people all over the world. If you or someone you love has an illness or you know that your body is not functioning properly, I urge you to learn more about the holistic approach to maintaining the health of your body.

After 50 years of resisting even aspirin and beginning in January of 2001, I ingested, at one or another, the following: Acyclovir, Ativan, ALG Rabbit Serum, Ambien, Attarax ATG Horse Serum, Benadryl, Cephapime, Celebrex, Cemethekone, Cymedadine, Cipro, Cyclophosphamide, Collate, Cytoxan, CYCLOSPORINE, Demerol, Desferol, Diflucan, Epogen/Procrit, Folic Acid, GCF, GSF, Halycion, Hydrocortisone, IL-11, Magnesium, Milk of Magnesia, Morphine, Neupogen, Penicillin, Pentamidine, Pepcid, Prednisone, Prednisone, Prilosec, Procrit/Epogin, Protonic, Solumedrol, Simethicone, Tagamet, Tylenol, and Vancomycin. And I was getting sicker by the day!

On July 9th of that year, I discontinued all drugs and launched my personal wellness plan primarily based on nutritional healing and am happy to report that as of September 8, 2002, I am golfing five days per week, visiting with my grandchild, walking, talking and taking out the trash.

I have not had a Red Blood Cell Transfusion since May 24 and have not needed a platelet transfusion since July 23. In the same timeframe of 2001, I was virtually flat on my back in a hospital bed and completely dependent on these transfusions to keep me alive.

I changed my lifestyle from type A to a much more relaxed approach, changed my diet from Mickey D's to "grains, greens and beans" and detoxified my body with a daily sauna and detox routine. I now eat only organically grown vegetables, lots of rice, beans and lettuces, drink only pure spring water, exercise 45-60 minutes per day and get at least 1-2 hours of sunshine every day.

During my recovery, I also took multivitamins, B12, Co-Q10, Vitamin E, Magnasorb, Essential Oils, Glutathione and a series of allergy and Alpha Lymphatic Factor shots developed specifically for me by the Environmental Health Center in Dallas, Texas. I now receive virtually all my nutrients from natural sources.

For the first fifty years of my life, I ignored the danger signals my body was sending me. With my new approach I fully expect good health for the next fifty. It is never too late to adopt a personal wellness plan of your own. See you on the other side!

And now with the second edition, it has been 18 years since my first trip to the Emergency Room where I met Doctor Kirshner and the incredible journey began.

Sincerely,
Bruce Lande 1/9/2019

www.ingramcontent.com/pod-product-compliance
Lightning Source LLC
Chambersburg PA
CBHW030606220526
45463CB00004B/1184